COMPUTER SCIENCE, TECHNOLOGY AND APPLICATIONS

MEDICAL KNOWLEDGE EXTRACTION FROM BIG DATA

Computer Science, Technology and Applications

Additional books and e-books in this series can be found on Nova's website under the Series tab.

COMPUTER SCIENCE, TECHNOLOGY AND APPLICATIONS

MEDICAL KNOWLEDGE EXTRACTION FROM BIG DATA

CONSTANTINOS M. KOUTSOJANNIS
EDITOR

nova
science publishers
New York

Library of Congress Cataloging-in-Publication Data

ISBN: 978-1-53617-925-5
Names: Koutsojannis, Constantinos, editor.
Title: Medical knowledge extraction from big data / Constantinos M. Koutsojannis, editor. Description: New York : Nova Science Publishers, [2020] | Series: Computer science, technology and applications | Includes bibliographical references and index. | Summary: "Data mining refers to the activity of going through big data sets to look for relevant information. As human health care data are the most difficult of all data to collect and their primary direction is the treatment of patients, and secondarily dealing with research, almost the only vindication for collecting medical data is to benefit the disease. All data miners should take into account that Medical Knowledge Extraction is internally connected with the Evidence-Based Medical approach because it uses data for already treated or not patients and there are times that opposites to Guideline Based medical practice. Additonally all researchers should be aware when are dealing with medical databases they may face the possibility that their work will never be accepted or even used from health care professionals if all these obligations will not be correctly addressed from the early beginning. In the present book, one can find after the three introductory chapters, a number of successfully evaluated applications that have been developed after mining approaches in Big or smaller amount (according to the application) of medical Data in different fields of every day clinical practice from teams of experts. The challenging adventure of Medical Knowledge Extraction can be followed by ambitious researchers finally resulting in a successful decision support system, that sometimes is so novel that it will provide new directions for basic or clinical research further that the existed. At least this procedure will save the experience of the best doctors on duty and will help young residents to be better and better"-- Provided by publisher. Identifiers: LCCN 2020018260 (print) | LCCN 2020018261 (ebook) | ISBN 9781536179255 (paperback) | ISBN 9781536179262 (adobe pdf) Subjects: LCSH: Medicine--Data processing. | Data mining. | Big data. Classification: LCC R858 .M3974 2020 (print) | LCC R858 (ebook) | DDC 610.285--dc23
LC record available at https://lccn.loc.gov/2020018260
LC ebook record available at https://lccn.loc.gov/2020018261

Published by Nova Science Publishers, Inc. † New York

To my
Spiritual father
Kyrillos

Contents

PREFACE

Big data and data mining are two different things, as the two terms are used for two different elements of the same kind of computer operation. Big data is a term for a large data set. Big data sets are those that outgrow the simple kind of database and data handling architectures that were used in earlier times when big data was more expensive.

Data mining refers to the activity of going through big data sets to look for relevant information. The general concept is that databases collect massive sets of data that may be homogeneous or automatically collected. Decision-makers need access to smaller, more specific pieces of data from those large sets. They use data mining for knowledge extraction that means to uncover the pieces of information that can help in decision making.

Human health care data are the most difficult of all data to collect, deal and analyze. As in medicine the primary direction is the care work for a specific patient, and secondarily dealing with him as researching resources; almost the only vindication for collecting medical data is to benefit the aforementioned individual disease.

The first important issue is that software engineers or researchers that are working in other fields will never face the same constraints of primarily *privacy-sensitive*, greatly heterogeneous, and massive medical data. Consequently, after prepossessing and cleaning parts, they will finally deal with just a small group of data that is the real treasure!

The second important issue is that most of the health care data have particular obligations concerning their *openness* to other people that are not dealing with the specific patient; their emergency (often dealing with life and death); and the ethical commitment to be used only for salutary. Consequently, all researchers should be aware when are dealing with medical databases they may face the possibility that their work will never be accepted or even used from health care professionals if all these obligations will not be correctly addressed from the early beginning.

The last but not the least important is the *transparency* of medical knowledge extracted from big medical databases is the *holy grail*, for pure knights of science searching for the truth resulting from the appropriate acceptancy from end-users as medical community members. Additionally, all data miners should take into account that Medical Knowledge Extraction is internally connected with the Evidence-Based Medical approach because it uses data for already treated or not patients and there are times that opposites to Guideline Based medical practice.

In the present book, one can find after the three introductory chapters, a number of successfully evaluated applications that have been developed after medical Big or smaller (according to the application) data mining approaches in different fields of every day clinical practice from teams of experts. The challenging adventure of Medical Knowledge Extraction can be followed by ambitious researchers finally resulting in a successful decision support system, that some times is so novel that it will provide new directions for basic or clinical research further that the existed! At least this procedure will save the experience of the best doctors on duty and will help young residents to be better and better.

I wish to express my appreciation to all authors-members of my Health Physics and Computational Intelligence Laboratory, as well as all other collaborating Laboratories and Departments of my University, for their friendship and willingness to share their deep knowledge and experience on the field. I wish most of them to feel more and more the happiness of a successful system that will in the future store more effectively the precious experience of our best doctors!

It is my pleasure to acknowledge my institute, University of Patras and all my colleagues including professors, from other departments, MSc students and staff that have supported me in this effort.

Additionally, I would like to repeatedly express to my wife, Maria that I am deeply indebted to her love and support all these years.

Finally I would like to underline my lifelong respect to my spiritual father *Kyrillos Kostopoulos* who is the main responsible for whatever possibly good I am today, and specifically for his blessing and his pray from the very beginning of my scientific and academic route.

Constantinos M Koutsojannis

Patras,
Hellas

In: Medical Knowledge Extraction ... ISBN: 978-1-53617-925-5
Editor: C. M. Koutsojannis

Chapter 1

MEDICAL BIG DATA

Anthi Malliori**, PhD
Department of Medical Physics, University Patras, Patras, Greece

ABSTRACT

The rapid growth of digital data brings substantial changes but also new potentials in many fields. Big data characterized commonly using four elements -volume, variety, velocity, veracity, can prove extremely beneficial on making associations and revealing hidden information. The healthcare sector is currently witnessing substantial advancements using such insights derived from big data in clinical applications and biomedical research. A wide range of functions, from data management to disease prediction and discovery of new drugs have considerably benefited from the emerging big data technologies and applications. Apart from the opportunities, challenges have also incurred commonly met when dealing with the scale and diversity of big data but also related to the special nature of medical data. Issues such as access, privacy, data ownership, reliability need to be addressed. The implementation of innovative tools is necessary to enable research using big data focus on aspects like predictive and personalized medicine in the future. Additional steps also need to be made facing the upcoming limitations, so that big data in healthcare can reach their full potential.

*Corresponding Author's Email: anmall@upatras.gr.

Keywords: big data, healthcare, data mining, biomedical research

INTRODUCTION

The Science of Big Data

Big Data and big data analytics are moving firmly in many fields. Along with Internet of Things (IoT) facilitating the easy and fast collection and exchange of the data, Cloud Computing and advances in Data Mining methods, they enable everyday services and applications to be converted into 'smart' technologies defining new eras in academia, industry, and government [1]. The potential of 'extracting meaning from big data' i.e., discovering associations, patterns, and trends within them, holds the promise of evolving aspects such as management and strategic decision making in more intelligent, effective and cost-efficient ways. More and more companies and organizations are adopting data-driven models and big data applications in an attempt to extract insights that will lead to better decisions and to a competitive advantage in their field [2].

Prior to big data, the estimations were mainly based on sampling data using a statistical analysis approach. Although, even small samples can result in high levels of accuracy for predictions and are considered to sufficiently represent the entire dataset, the benefits of using vast quantities of information give big data the lead [3]. Using more data and in some cases, all the data about a phenomenon could reveal details that we would never be able to see before. Even with big data being characterized as 'messy' and of generally lower quality compared to data carefully collected by researchers, the big volume is still considered to outweigh 'cleaner' but fewer data [4]. Moreover, in cases where the volume of big data is combined with very high quality i.e., such as the data produced in genomic analysis, their predictive power scales up. Unlike traditional data, the term big data refers not only to large growing data sets but also heterogeneous data types and formats that had not been considered together until now. Due to the size and the complex nature of these data streams, it is difficult -

or even impossible- to be managed with common tools, thus powerful technologies and advanced data models, algorithms and architectures are required. In this framework, advancements such as optimization of parallel programming and low-level languages, data storage solutions and new database technologies, new -often nonlinear- tools for data analysis have been developed.

Big data benefit a lot from processing methods based on Artificial Intelligence (AI). Machine Learning (ML) algorithms are widely used to 'train' machines perform certain tasks by learning complex relationships or patterns from large amounts of empirical data [5]. Contrary to conventional algorithms that usually involve rows of code with specific instructions, in ML it is the data that act as examples so that machines can learn from experience. Therefore, the huge amounts of data facilitate the training and enable machines to constantly auto-improve as the available data increase. The applications are not only limited to everyday decision-making processes as these algorithms can also have a great impact on long-term strategies and support extensive and high-quality research in every domain. Ranging from behavioral patterns and purchasing trends to medical applications such as diagnoses and treatment models [6, 7], big data can play a key role including advantages and potential barriers. Scientists in each field are aided to better understand the mechanisms and functions beneath the facts, foresee the progression of different situations, improve predictive models, create more sophisticated and advanced decision support systems but also have to face the challenges that come along.

Types of Big Data

Big data offer information whose scale and diversity give a new potential in representing the real world. International Data Corporation (IDC) estimated the size of the 'digital universe' to be 40,000 exabytes (EB) or 40 zettabytes (ZB) by 2020 [8]. Big data can be found in the form of structured or unstructured data. A third category is also possibly known as semi-structured data or data with the self-describing structure which are considerably easier to analyze compared to the unstructured ones.

i Structured

Structured data are considered the most 'traditional' type of data storage, since the earliest versions of database management systems (DBMS) and have a familiar, fixed format well-known in advance. These data can be stored, recalled and analyzed easily, as they conform to a predefined model that is straightforward to process. Due to this model, data from each field can be accessed separately or in combination with data from other fields, speeding up the procedures and adding a major strength to this type of data. Structured data have a tabular format with common examples being excel files or SQL databases. Although there have been several techniques developed for working with such data, in the case of big data where the size grows to a huge extent, new challenges are involved in the storage and processing procedures.

ii Unstructured

Unstructured data have information that is not organized in a pre-defined form or structure typically originating from heterogeneous sources. As a result, their processing is difficult using common programs compared to the cases where structured databases are involved. In addition to the unknown model, the huge size of big data makes it extremely challenging to extract values out of them. Typical examples of unstructured data may involve audio, images, video files, simple text files or No-SQL databases. New available technologies and tools specialized for this type of data have enhanced the ability for their storing and processing.

iii Semi-Structured

Semi-structured data is a third category, lying in between the other two types of big data. Their form is not conforming to the formal structure of data models from relational databases or other well-known formats. In fact, they could be considered unstructured if it weren't for the tags that are contained within them. These keywords act as markers and help to differentiate important elements and create some hierarchies and grouping. The most common examples of semi-structured data are XML files and JavaScript Object Notation (JSON). Emails could also be considered in this category due to their native meta-data that enables classification and keyword indexing without any additional tools.

Characteristics - 'The 4 V's'

Big data represent amounts of data, which according to the definition given by D. Laney, are growing in three different primary dimensions - *volume, velocity,* and *variety* [9]. A fourth characteristic - *veracity*, representing the uncertainty or degree of credibility of the data has been also introduced over time [10, 11], making the combination of all these elements, known as 'the 4 V's' (Figure 1), a typical and indicative representation of the nature of big data.

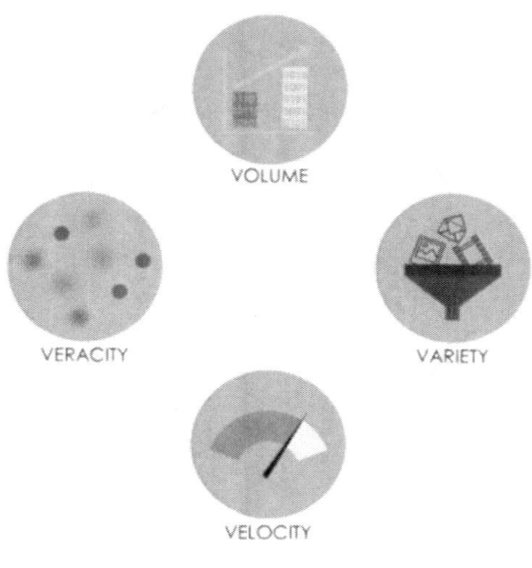

Figure 1. Characteristics of Big Data.

i Volume

Volume is the first characteristic of big data. Data are generated continuously and their already huge volume is expected to increase even more with extremely fast rates in the years to come. In the big data context, it is essential to realize the crucial role of size in extracting value out of them and thus to deal with the challenges coming with it. Consequently, appropriate storage and mining methods are necessary to be developed.

ii Variety

Variety indicates the significant heterogeneity that exists among the available datasets due to the different sources and nature of the stored data ranging from unstructured and structured texts, signals, images and videos to numerical data and meta-data. Moreover, the continuously growing data streams available from emails, big databases, social media or other sources make the management of the diversity of big data as complex as dealing with their huge volume and triggers the need for advanced pre- and post-processing analytics.

iii Velocity

Velocity refers to the rate of data collection and the speed of analytical processing and thus the availability of the outputs and insights for decision making. Since the flow of data is constant and rapid, their fast interpretation could exploit the full potential of big data and revolutionize specific fields such as healthcare, with future real-time applications detecting incidents as early as possible and pointing towards the right treatments [10].

iv Veracity

Veracity is indicative up to which extent big data, and thus the derived outcomes, are error-free and reliable. Due to the big variety in the sources and conditions during data collection, the need for such an element representing the credibility of the data is high. Especially in the healthcare sector, data quality issues are crucial and deriving the accurate data from different record files or real signals through a 'noisy' environment, could be challenging.

BIG DATA IN HEALTHCARE

Promises

Medical big data following the general concept are also characterized by 'the 4 V's' with massive amounts of generated data coming mainly from electronic health records (EHR), radiology images, biomedical signals, clinical trials as well as newer forms of data i.e., 3D imaging, genomics, data from biometric sensors. The diversity in the nature of the collected data along with the speed that they are generated during routine healthcare and biomedical research, pose new challenges but also hold great promise for clinical applications and new discoveries [12].

Areas ranging from epidemiology and research to primary clinical care could benefit much from applications, such as personal monitoring, early diagnosis, clinical decision support [13]. Big data analytics can make associations even in lack of full evidence in cases where answers cannot be found through conventional methods. The extraction of information and possible patterns from big data, a term is known as 'data mining', is widely applied giving access to otherwise missing knowledge. Such algorithms have the potential to provide healthcare professionals with models related to the occurrence and evolvement of certain medical conditions including complicated neurodegenerative disorders [14, 15] or even prediction of cancer and drug responses [16, 17]. Insights on possible treatment outcomes could be extremely valuable in clinical practice for accurate decision making.

It is widely known that biological systems, such as human cells, are systems of great complexity, combining molecular and physical phenomena with interactions that need to be deeply understood in order to be studied thoroughly. The major advantage of big data in finding correlations and revealing hidden patterns among them could be very helpful for researchers in better understanding the biological processes, resulting in tremendous opportunities for prognosis and breakthrough treatments in the future. Moreover, combining genomic data with data from EHR and other clinical information leads to a more thorough description of the individual patient profile and brings one step closer to what is called 'precision or personalized medicine' [8].

The reduction of waste in resources is another big issue in the healthcare sector. Although there are many efforts towards this direction, there is still much that could be done to optimize patient outcomes and at the same time better control the healthcare costs. Efficient exploitation of the insights of big data coming from everyday practice and scientific research could gradually improve quality in healthcare and the existing gap between costs and outcomes, leading to a 'continuous learning healthcare system' [13].

Big Data technologies have also brought changes to pharma companies trying to adopt smart solutions. Drugs and devices with advanced sensors will be able to collect data for further analysis improving personal care [18] while insights from safety report databases will enable the identification of drug associations and risk factors [19]. New possibilities are created for personalized treatments and advanced services, fewer adverse drug effects, disease surveillance [11, 20], medical device safety and vigilance [13].

Challenges

Big data apart from the advantages and promises have many challenges to face, related to their characteristics and especially their large volume and heterogeneity. There is a need for new technologies, mainly based on parallel processing approaches and cloud-based storage, to be able to handle the vast amounts of information and make them easily accessible to the scientific community. In addition to this, the development of new bioinformatic-based tools and the involvement of multidisciplinary experts are necessary in order to deal with the diversity of information and end up in unified formats. Furthermore, supporting real-time analytics and 'cleaning' of data are also challenges that have to be dealt with, in most fields using big data and especially in healthcare [8].

Medical big data -due to their nature- have also some distinctive characteristics, creating special challenges that need to be separately and successfully addressed. An important feature, for example, is that decision making should be fully justified, keeping up with the high safety context of medical practice [13]. Decision algorithms are frequently considered as 'black boxes' by the medical community and they are often hard to be accepted. Moreover, medical data are not easily accessed and most healthcare professionals and researchers are reluctant to data sharing and generally to the open data concept [21]. Data ownership issues and patient privacy concerns make accessibility even harder. This obstructs reproducibility and limits the sharing of medical knowledge. Even with all the new methods developed and the technological advancements, there is a still relatively small number of research findings that have been transferred to clinical practice.

Another obstacle is the missing details from the clinical data stored in the EHR [8, 12]. In most cases, details concerning the partial outcomes throughout the patient therapy are not available, as EHR was primarily designed to facilitate administrative and management purposes rather than scientific research. As a result, information concerning the progress of a disease in relation to the various therapeutic schemes may not be easily extracted from these data. Similar reasons for missing data may exist in the difficulty to transfer all the useful information from handwritten reports or errors induced during this procedure.

Despite the generally huge volume of big data, the volume of medical big data could be characterized as relatively small, considering other disciplines, and there are still reasons that could further limit the size of the set that will be finally used. For example, due to filters and selection criteria that are most of the time imposed for specific research purposes, it is possible that very few cases may return from queries in the end. As a result, the small cohort restrains statistical confidence even for the case of widely used databases with data of thousands of patients, such as MIMIC III [12]. In addition to this, possible errors and missing information during data transfer from reports may induce a degree of uncertainty to the collected data.

CURRENT STATUS AND FUTURE PROSPECTS

Developed Applications, Platforms, and Bioinformatics Tools

Medical big data analytics are increasingly earning their special place in today's healthcare sector. Various open-source applications have been developed for storing, distributing and parallel processing of complex big data. One of the most popular platforms for such purposes is Hadoop [22]. Hadoop is based on the principles of mapping and reducing operations while at the same time is able to handle failures efficiently, providing high-quality services. Appache Spark [23] is another option for the management of big data. Appache, exploits in-memory data computing resulting in much faster processing compared to Hadoop for small datasets (especially when data size does not exceed available memory). A promising source of medical big data is the so-called 'omics' data. Large-scale genetic sequencing studies have grown huge expectations and led to the development of several tools for the analysis of such data. Among them, DistMap, CloudBurst, and BlueSNP are some of the widely used applications based on the Hadoop framework for mapping reads and efficiently handling sequencing data [24].

The growing demands in this field, have led over the past few years, to the implementation of integrated commercial platforms dedicated to healthcare big data analytics. Companies such as IBM Corporation, Ayasdi, Flatiron Health have developed platforms incorporating methods based on AI, for the analysis of the medical data. Similarly, other big companies like Oracle Corporation and Google Inc., are also moving towards this direction. These commercial solutions focus on uncovering important insights and providing innovative outcomes in healthcare. Ayasdi for example, among others, uses AI methods for assessment of population health, risk management and selection of proactive strategies. IBM Watson Health is a platform integrating AI technologies, that aims to extract the maximum possible information from the available sources. The main goals are to provide services on sharing clinical data among hospitals and assist advance research, especially studies related to cancer disease models and treatment options.

A subcategory of AI is the ML algorithms. These algorithms can be used for information extraction from images (ML methods can extract structured information out of them). Moreover, available developed software such as Optical Character Recognition (OCR), can digitize information by turning images into 'machine-readable' text and thus enrich EHRs with the information included in hand-written notes from patient histories and data [8]. Medical images contain patient data of large sizes that can be used for analysis, diagnosis, predictions, and decision making support. Current ML algorithms particularly focus on the extraction of unstructured or hidden information existing in such clinical images. These data might not be easily observed otherwise, and can enhance diagnostic capability i.e., extract insights on disease-related biomarkers or monitor new treatments.

Several software tools have been developed for medical image analytics with most of them supporting multiple input types and functions. For instance, GIMIAS and Elastix can be used to perform registration, visualization, reconstruction, simulation and diffusion to extract information from a wide range of inputs (MRI, Ultrasound, X-Ray, fMRI, PET, CT-Scan, EEG, Mammogram) [25, 26]. Similarly, there is software for analyzing medical 3D images such as Visualization Toolkit (VTK) provided by Kitware, Inc. [27] and Medical Imaging Interaction Toolkit (MITK)[28]. Statistical Parametric Mapping (SPM) [29], is another tool developed by the Wellcome Department of Imaging Neuroscience (University College London). It was primarily used for the analysis of brain image data sequences, having the ability to process images of different types i.e., fMRI, PET, SPECT, aiming to identify brain responses and characterize disease-related changes.

CONCLUSION AND FUTURE PROSPECTS

The exponential growth of medical big data has changed the potential and grown many expectations in the healthcare sector. Several aspects in clinical care can be supported, including among other personal monitoring, early diagnosis, decision making. Big data in combination with ML methods finding patterns and making correlations among data from genomics, medical images or other forms of patient clinical data can prove extremely valuable in biomedical research. The possibility of extracting meaning and revealing otherwise hidden information out of big data is very promising for disease prognosis and the discovery of new treatments. Close monitoring and analysis of information coming from healthcare big data can optimize patient outcomes and lead to improved ways of data management. More efficient control of healthcare costs can be achieved reducing waste in resources. Finally, providing insights from safety report databases can help towards further improvement of medical devices and the reduction of adverse drug effects. Apart from the great opportunities arising, many constraints related to the nature of medical big data have also come up. Challenges created from heterogeneity, speed of the generated and collected data, as well as their often characterization as 'messy' and of generally lower quality, have been addressed. Issues such as reliability and acceptance of ML methods and decision-making algorithms, missing data and errors induced during the transfer of useful patient record details have been discussed, posing credibility questions for the use of big data. Additionally, selection criteria that are often used with queries in available patient datasets may further narrow the finally used set of data limiting the statistical significance. Moreover, access, privacy, and data ownership issues have been reported. All the above-mentioned restrictions hold back the adoption of the results coming from big data and result in a limited transfer of research findings to clinical practice.

Overall, it appears that the use of big data has created extremely promising opportunities for healthcare up to now, there are still additional steps to be made in the future though. Among the already developed tools, several platforms are available enabling storing, distributing and fast processing of big data. Additionally, software focusing on analyzing and extracting information out of medical images has been implemented supporting multiple inputs and functions as well as algorithms based on ML suitable for simulations and diagnostic modeling. However, much more should be done in this direction. Specifically, there is a need for the development of innovative diagnostic tools based on sophisticated models of the human body with detailed integrated information coming from both physiological and –omic data. Future research should focus on insights coming from big data, for the discovery of new biomarkers and therapeutic interventions. Another aspect to be pointed out is the need to focus on predictive medicine. Advanced models can provide valuable information concerning the evolvement of a disease or can even enable the prognosis of a situation. Data related to the healthy population can help in the prediction of epidemics delivering early warnings and providing information on the disease. A final point to be emphasized is the opportunity big data can offer towards a transition to more personalized medical treatments. In a world of constantly increasing data, big data analysis and the subsequent insights will continue playing a crucial role. It is critical to find solutions to the emerging challenges and to further develop this new promising era in the future, exploiting the full potential of big data for the benefit of healthcare.

References

[1] Zanella, A., et al., *Internet of things for smart cities.* IEEE Internet of Things J, 2014. 1(1): p. 22-32.

[2] Stucke, M. and A. Grunes, *Big Data and Competition Policy*. 2016: Oxford University Press.

[3] Hansen, M.M., et al., *Big Data in Science and Healthcare: A Review of Recent Literature and Perspectives. Contribution of the IMIA Social Media Working Group.* Yearb Med. Inform., 2014. 9: p. 21-6.
[4] Mayer-Schönberger, V. and K. Cuckie, *Big Data: A Revolution that Will Transform how We Live, Work, and Think.* 2013: Houghton Mifflin Harcourt. Chapter 2.
[5] Bishop, C.M., *Pattern recognition and machine learning.* Information science and statistics. 2006, New York: Springer. xx, 738 p.
[6] Jones, L.D., et al., *Artificial intelligence, machine learning and the evolution of healthcare: A bright future or cause for concern? Bone Joint Res.*, 2018. 7(3): p. 223-225.
[7] Wang, S. and R.M. Summers, *Machine learning and radiology. Med. Image Anal.*, 2012. 16(5): p. 933-51.
[8] Dash, S., et al., *Big data in healthcare: management, analysis and future prospects. Journal of Big Data*, 2019. 6(1).
[9] Laney, D., *3D Data Management: Controlling Data Volume, Velocity and Variety. META Group Research Note*, 6, 2001.
[10] Raghupathi, W. and V. Raghupathi, *Big data analytics in healthcare: promise and potential. Health Inf. Sci. Syst.*, 2014. 2: p. 3.
[11] Bellazzi, R., *Big Data and Biomedical Informatics: A Challenging Opportunity. Yearbook of Medical Informatics*, 2018. 23(01): p. 08-13.
[12] Adibuzzaman, M., et al., *Big data in healthcare - the promises, challenges and opportunities from a research perspective: A case study with a model database. AMIA Annu. Symp. Proc.*, 2017: p. 384-392.
[13] Lee, C.H. and H.J. Yoon, *Medical big data: promise and challenges. Kidney Res. Clin. Pract.,* 2017. 36(1): p. 3-11.
[14] Megalooikonomou, V., et al., *Data mining in brain imaging.Stat. Methods Med. Res.,* 2000. 9(4): p. 359-94.
[15] Nayak, L., et al., *Computational neuroscience and neuroinformatics: Recent progress and resources. J. Biosci.,* 2018. 43(5): p. 1037-1054.

[16] Kourou, K., et al., *Machine learning applications in cancer prognosis and prediction. Comput. Struct. Biotechnol. J.*, 2015. 13: p. 8-17.

[17] Vougas, K., et al., *Machine learning and data mining frameworks for predicting drug response in cancer: An overview and a novel in silico screening process based on association rule mining. Pharmacol. Ther.,* 2019: p. 107395.

[18] Dimitrov, D.V., *Medical Internet of Things and Big Data in Healthcare.* H*ealthc Inform. Res.*, 2016. 22(3): p. 156-63.

[19] Ventola, C.L., *Big Data and Pharmacovigilance: Data Mining for Adverse Drug Events and Interactions.* P T, 2018. 43(6): p. 340-351.

[20] Hay, S.I., et al., *Big data opportunities for global infectious disease surveillance. PLoS Med.*, 2013. 10(4): p. e1001413.

[21] Scruggs, S.B., et al., *Harnessing the heart of big data.Circ. Res.*, 2015. 116(7): p. 1115-9.

[22] Shvachko, K., et al., *The Hadoop Distributed File System*, in *2010 IEEE 26th Symposium on Mass Storage Systems and Technologies (MSST)*. 2010. p. 1-10.

[23] *The Apache Software Foundation. Apache Spark. Wilmington, DE.* 2015.

[24] Tripathi, R., et al., *Next-generation sequencing revolution through big data analytics. Frontiers in Life Science* 2016. 9(2): p. 119-149

[25] *GIMIAS (http://www.gimias.org/).*

[26] *elastix (http://elastix.isi.uu.nl/).*

[27] Schroeder, W., K. Martin, and B. Lorensen, *The visualization toolkit: An Object-Oriented Approach to 3D Graphics*. 4th ed. 2006: Kitware. 528 p.

[28] Wolf, I., et al., *The medical imaging interaction toolkit.* Med.*Image Anal.*, 2005. 9(6): p. 594-604.

[29] Friston, K.J., *Statistical parametric mapping : the analysis of funtional brain images*. 1st ed. 2007, Amsterdam; Boston: Elsevier/Academic Press. 647 p.

BIOGRAPHICAL SKETCH

Anthi Malliori

Anthi Malliori was born in 1983 in Patras. She received her dipoma in Electrical and Computer Engineering in 2007 at the University of Patras, Greece. During 2007-2008, she attended the MSc in Biomedical Engineering and Medical Imaging at the University College London, UK and received the UCL Alumni Scholarship. In 2014, she received her PhD from the interdepartmental program in Biomedical Engineering (BME) organized by the Medical School of Patras and the National Technical University of Athens (NTUA), Greece under the Heraclitus II (2010-2013) research program. Currently, she is a researcher at the Biomedical Technology Unit, Laboratory of Medical Physics, University of Patras. She is teaching Medical Informatics, Orthotics-Prosthetics and Intelligent Decision Support Systems at Faculty of Health Rehabilitation Sciences at the University of Patras. Her research interests focus on Medical Imaging and Informatics and she is currently involved in a European project related to Smart devises and applications and a National project concerning Diagnosis Techniques using Machine Learning. She has published in several international journals and conferences in her research field.

In: Medical Knowledge Extraction ...
Editor: C. M. Koutsojannis
ISBN: 978-1-53617-925-5

Chapter 2

DATA MINING IN HEALTH SCIENCES

Andreas Andrikopoulos*
Laboratory of Health Physics & Computational Intelligence,
University of Patras, Patras, Greece

ABSTRACT

The evolution of technology has made it possible for the Internet to spread. As time went on, access to the Internet became more and more accessible to more and more people. This, in turn, has led to the development of more sites and the use of databases to store data. The creation of commercial and social websites has been the first step in the demands and needs for storing and managing large volumes of data. Today, the amount of data available is enormous and is growing exponentially every day. The reduction in the cost of collection and the difficulty in collecting and storing data contributed significantly to the development of this field. The huge amount of data that accumulates in databases and data warehouses cannot be exploited as it is. Some steps must first be taken to structure the data properly so that it can then be exploited. The state-of-the-art technology and the simultaneous rapid development and rapid expansion of communications lead to the provision and supply of information in every sphere of human activity.

* Corresponding Author's Email: anandrikop@gmail.com.

Today, digital media enables the continuous recording and storage of large amounts of data. The challenge is to manage and exploit this data in order to generate valuable knowledge and extract it for future use. A contemporary challenge that the database mining and discovery sector promise to serve. Especially today, in health sciences, the usefulness and necessity of health data mining services are being discussed and experts as a whole converge on these new technologies and practices should be gradually adopted. Health databases need to be extracted as content endless and complex data whose processing and analysis by non-automated manner becomes expensive and certainly not practical. The knowledge that can be gained on effective treatments or best practices is undoubtedly valuable and beneficial to both the practitioners and the patients themselves.

Keywords: data mining, information reliability, big data analytics, health sector

RECURSION AND EVOLUTION

Since the mid-1980s, there has been an unprecedented global explosion in the ability to produce, store and send data, mainly in digital form. Another development that is a component of this trend is the increased access to Information and Communication Technologies (ICT), which is made possible by personal computers, smartphones, and other mobile devices. These improved capabilities in terms of data storage, coupled with high-speed computing power as well as real-time information delivery over the Internet, have led to an exponential increase in the average daily data consumption of the individual [1]. In light of the significant increase in the data output, rapid digitization has taken place in all industries. This digital transformation has also taken place in the health sector in the form of increased use of both Electronic Medical Records (EMR) and Health Information Systems (HIS) and portable and smart devices. As a result, a huge amount and variety of digital health data are now available, which in addition to clinical data, includes biological data (-omics data), socio-demographic data or even insurance claims. Although these high-quality data are potential of increasing importance for optimizing healthcare provision, they are still perceived more as a by-product of healthcare provision and less as a central source of data critical to achieving competitive advantage in the sector. As electronic health data remains largely untapped, the need to convert processed data into useful and effective information is imperative [2].

The health sector has always been generating large volumes of data due to the increased need for record-keeping in the context of patient care [3]. Many of these available and highly valuable data are in unstructured or semi-structured form. Further, the complex, dynamic, and heterogeneous features of this data [4, 6] make it difficult to extract useful information through the use of traditional analytical tools and techniques. Thus, BigData (or Big Data) in the field of health is an important issue, not only because of its enormous volume but also because of the diversity of data and hence the speed of its management [4]. In fact, humans have a finite capacity to process this data and therefore effective decision support is needed. This creates the need to integrate Big Data Analytics into the health field [7]. Big Data Analytics has the ability to analyze a wide range of complex data and produce valuable information that otherwise would not be possible to extract. When applied to health data, they are able not only to identify emerging patterns but also to improve the quality of health care, reduce costs and make timely decisions [7]. As typically noted in the report of McKinsey International Institute [8], if BigData were to be used effectively, the US health care system would save more than $ 300 billion a year, two-thirds of which would be in the form of reduced health care costs. about 8%. Using BigData technology and the automated analysis of results, useful information can emerge that has remained obscure until recently [7].

Advances in cloud computing and the growing development of electronic medical records now allow easy access to timely patient data. Over time, integrating these longitudinal patient data with data from different, structured and unstructured BigData sources offers the opportunity to fully understand the diseases. The ability of BigDataAnalytics to detect disease heterogeneity allows not only their timely and accurate diagnosis but also the evaluation of existing therapies.

Through the 12th correlation of data from different sources and through the identification of various distinct patterns, the predictive power of BigDataAnalytics can also be exploited to convert continuous data into valuable real-time information. This capability provided by big data analytics is especially important in medical emergencies as it can judge the difference between life and death [7]. Storing and keeping BigData in the health sector promises to improve the quality of healthcare while reducing costs. Among other things, it has the potential to support various functions performed in the context of medical and health care, including clinical decision support, epidemiological surveillance, and population health management. Reportedly, health data maintained in the US alone exceeds 150 exabytes (10^{18}bytes) in 2011 and has the potential to exceed even larger size ranges such as zettabytes (10^{21}bytes) and yottabytes (10^{24}gigabytes). It is understood that due to the huge volume of BigData, their analysis is a real issue. Therefore, health professionals are seeking the help of computer science to explore and find solutions to convert data into information and knowledge [2].

The rapidly expanding BigDataAnalytics sector is beginning to play a central role in the evolution of health practices and research. In particular, Big Data Analytics has provided tools for the accumulation, management, analysis and assimilation of large volumes of different, structured and structured data generated by current healthcare systems. However, despite its remarkable outlook in terms of improving health care provision and a greater understanding of diseases, the adoption and development of research in this area still lag behind and are hampered by some of the key problems inherent in the BigData thematic [9]. The promising value of BigData technology in the field of health has created a growing interest among researchers in the academic and industrial communities. However, a limited number of relevant reviews can be identified, and international literature remains largely fragmented [7].

Main Features of Big Data in the Health Sector

The volume of health data is expected to increase dramatically in the future and it is, therefore, becoming clear that the need to find new and intelligent ways of managing data is more urgent than ever. Health is one of those sectors where huge volumes of data and information are generated and consumed per second, and therefore no one could question the importance of optimizing them in order to draw valuable conclusions. Another development concerns the compensation models of healthcare providers changing. The effective use of health services and pay for performance are emerging as new critical factors in today' s healthcare environment. While profit is not and should not be their primary motivation, it is vital for health care organizations to have the tools, infrastructure, and techniques available to effectively leverage Big Data. Otherwise, they risk losing huge amounts of lost revenue and profits [3]. In addition, the rapid increase in health data has led to a shift in focus from treatment to disease prevention. Scientists have focused on improving the reliability and effectiveness of health care systems to minimize treatment costs, as well as providing better medicines to patients. Hospitals and national health systems are a rich BigData reservoir, including patient history files, clinical trial results, and imaging tests [14].

Existing analytical techniques can be applied to the enormous amount of existing (but not yet sufficiently analyzed) all kinds of medical data in order to gain a deeper understanding of the results, which will then be transferred and applied to the point of care. Ideally, knowledge of the population, as well as the individual themselves, will support and provide valuable information to the attending physician and patient throughout the decision-making process and facilitate the choice of the most appropriate therapeutic option for the particular patient[4]. Health is a great example of how BigData' s three definitions, namely speed, variety and volume, are an intrinsic aspect of the data it generates. These data are disseminated across multiple healthcare systems, insurance funds, researchers, government agencies, etc. In addition, each of these data repositories is overloaded and inherently unable to provide a platform that is transparent worldwide. In addition, an important addition to the above is the concept of validity, since the reliability of health data is also important for their effective use in the development of transcriptional research [4, 7].

Big data in healthcare is an important issue, not only because of the volume but also because of the variety of data types and the speed with which these data should be managed. Increased use of telemedicine will further test patient data storage capacity, and innovative use of GoogleGlass by physicians will also come to add to the social and behavioral aspects of BigData. Electronic medical records (EMRs) contain a wealth of data, such as patient demographics and clinical and genomic data, and are known to significantly support the good flow of healthcare [1]. Future real-time data applications, such as early detection of infections, timely identification, and administration of appropriate therapies could reduce patient morbidity and mortality and even prevent intra-hospital infections. Already, real-time streaming data is being used to monitor newborns in the Intensive Care Unit (ICU), alerting physicians to possible infections that threaten the life of the hospitalized neonate. The ability to perform large volume data analyzes across all specialties and in real-time will undoubtedly revolutionize health [15].

Healthcare data can be classified as structured, semi-structured or unstructured [3, 7, 12]. Structured data is data that can be easily stored, retrieved, retrieved, analyzed and manipulated by a computer program [3]. As mentioned above, structured data includes laboratory data, clinical sensor data and relational databases [16], semi-organized data includes data stored in XML (ExtensibleMarkupLanguage) interface. Unstructured data is free-text data that usually does not have a specific design and usually includes electronic medical records [12], handwritten notes, graphs, radiographs, patient discharge summaries, physiological measurements, health data from social media networking and smartphones [17]. 90% of BigData Health is in the form of unstructured data [12].

Already, new streams of data - both structured and unstructured - are crossing the health field, coming from fitness equipment, genetic and genomic studies, online research and other sources. However, data that can be read, stored and organized so that it can be processed by computer systems and analyzed for useful information is limited. In particular, health-related applications should have more efficient ways of combining and converting heterogeneous data, including modification from structured to unstructured data [3]. The characteristics of medical data contributing to their complexity include the diversity of different diseases and their comorbidities, heterogeneity of treatments and outcomes, differences in clinical workflows, different patterns of medical and nursing practice, patient populations, available technologies, and referral mechanisms [7]. However, big data analytics can overcome these issues as it is used for large-scale analysis and decision-making at a low cost. On the other hand, the gap between health care costs and health outcomes is one of the major issues and many developed countries are making significant efforts to close it. According to estimates, this gap is a common component of poor management of research results, limited utilization of available data, limited experience, which together has led to lost opportunities, wasted resources and potential harm to patients [1]

Big Data Health Perspectives

Healthcare data is disorganized and fragmented, comes from different sources and has different structures and forms [1, 7]. Clinical data, such as vital signs, patient medical history, medications, immunizations, and imaging tests, can be accessed from electronic health records, medical order entry systems (CPOE), clinical decision support systems (CDSS), records medication administration, laboratory and pharmaceutical records [3, 18] cohort studies, government investigations and clinical trials. On the other hand, the administrative data contain patient demographics and information from their visits to their doctor, the date of the patient's admission, the date he was discharged, the diagnosis during the International Statistical Classification of Diseases and Related Problems. Health (ICD), the patient's health status at discharge as well as financial requirements data including visitation fees, who should it pays the patient's health service fee as well as the health care provider's compensation [7, 18].

BigData sources in healthcare can be broadly classified as internal (eg health electronic records, clinical decision support systems, CPOEs, etc.) and external (government sources, laboratories, pharmacies, insurance companies, etc.). This data is held in multiple formats (flat files, relational tables, ASCII/texts, etc.), stored in multiple locations (both in terms of geographical location and in the sense that they are hosted on the premises of different healthcare providers), and are also observed in different applications (transaction processing applications, databases, etc.) [1]. From the above, it appears that BigData in Health includes data on physiology, behavior, molecular, clinical practice, environmental exposure, medical imaging, disease management, prescription medication history, diet or even exercise parameters. [19, 20]. In the international literature, there is no widely accepted classification of BigData sources in healthcare. One view identifies two major BigData sources, namely genomic research (genome-wide, gene expression, and sequencing data) and the buyer-provider of health services (data from electronic health records, insurance records, medication prescriptions, patient feedback, etc.) [7]. Key areas of health care that have benefited from Big Data include disease prevention, identifying modifiable risk factors for both, as well as planning interventions for changing one's behavior [1]. As reported by Rumsfeldetal. [20] BigData analysis in the field of health can contribute significantly to the following:

- Developing predictive models for risks and resource use
- Population management
- Supervision of medicines and technological safety
- Heterogeneity of diseases and treatments
- Precision medicine and clinical decision support systems
- Quality of care and performance measurement
- Public health

The digitization, correlation and efficient exploitation of Big Data brings with it a number of significant benefits for the whole spectrum of healthcare organizations, ranging from private practice to large hospital networks [21]. Possible benefits include detecting diseases at earlier stages, when they can be simpler and more efficiently managed, managing both the individual and the population's health, as well as timely and effective detection of healthcare fraud. Many questions may also be addressed by analyzing this data, which is a distinct scientific field: Big Data Analytics. Some developments or outcomes can be predicted or even calculated on the basis of a huge amount of historical data, such as duration of hospitalization (LOS), patients who choose to undergo elective surgery, patients who may not want to undergo surgery, complications, those at risk of developing medical complications, patients at risk of sepsis, inpatient illnesses, disease progression, and causative factors as well as concomitant diseases [3, 8]. Big data could reduce the so-called modernist bias. Modernist prejudice existed when recent events are considered more important and valid than previous events. However, it should be noted that especially in the field of health, innovative bias can lead to wrong decisions. In addition, in healthcare, Big Data is also used in predictive analysis, which focuses on identifying and addressing a medical issue before it becomes uncontrolled. Thus, by using information derived from processed Big Data, healthcare professionals can reduce the risk and overcome the problem at its birth [22]. The above analysis shows that, in order to improve the quality of health care and patient outcomes, there is an urgent need to increase both the availability of data and their analytical capabilities, factors that are commonly considered as central forces for of big data in the field of health [1].

BIG DATA ANALYTICS IN HEALTH

According to Peter Sondergaard saying, "*Information is the fuel of the 21st century and their analysis is the engine*." The data collected in various repositories by various organizations, as well as data produced by individuals can only make a difference if in other words, without proper analysis, the data will simply be a resource for the organization, but it is not exploited. The data sets are large and complex, posing enormous challenges to existing techniques that attempt to analyze and record results and possible correlations [11]. One term that is widely used today is Big Data Analytics. It is a process of transforming raw data into information. This substantive term describes the need to draw valuable conclusions and forecasts from the data, with the aim of helping decision-making and improving the processes of individual organizations [13]. To support decision-making in the fast-growing business, Big Data Analytics manages to uncover hidden patterns, identify relationships, understand market trends, customer preferences, and derive other useful business information.

Health Data Analytics or Health Analytics could be defined as systematic use of medical data and relevant management information through the application of analytical methods and tools, as well as quantitative and qualitative statistics, environmental analysis and forecasts, which may constitute a basis for action, as well as for the development of an information-based strategy and operational management for better health care [24]. In addition, Health Data Analytics or Health Analytics is a business term that encompasses a wide range of Big Data business intelligence and analytics applications. This new concept is based on the availability and accessibility of data and information gathered through the good integration and interoperability of a wide range of health information systems, such as electronic medical records, image archiving and communication systems, laboratory information systems and labs. - healthcare data storage systems [24]. Moving in the same direction, researchers Frost & Sullivan [23] proposed the concept of Advanced Health Analytics.

Recently, the number of data sources in the health sector has grown rapidly as a result of the widespread use of sensor technologies for smartphones and mobile systems. Therefore, it is difficult to carry out an analysis of these data using traditional analytical methods deemed inappropriate for handling large volumes of heterogeneous medical data [25]. From this perspective, healthcare organizations are undergoing extensive data processing sustained through the exploitation of Big Data Analytics [24, 26]. Big Data Analytics includes heterogeneous data integration, data quality control, analysis, modeling, and interpretation and verification [27, 28]. The correlation between data sets, and the development of predictive models using data mining techniques [29]. Big Data Analytics in medicine and healthcare integrates the analysis of various scientific fields such as bioinformatics, medical imaging, sensor computing, medical computing, and health computing. The new knowledge that comes from big data analytics techniques is expected to bring enormous benefits to patients, clinicians, and health policymakers [27].

Over the last two decades, Data Analytics in Health has become an important scientific field for both researchers and healthcare professionals, reflecting the extent of management's information-driven influence on problem-solving and decision-making [30]. Health information systems are rapidly adopted worldwide, which will significantly increase the quantity and improve the quality of available health data. At the same time, breakthroughs have been made in analytical methods for analyzing vast amounts of data and acquiring new knowledge. Consequently, there are no previous opportunities for using such methods to improve quality and reduce health care costs [24, 31].

BIG DATA ANALYTICS CLASSIFICATION IN HEALTH

The BigDataAnalytics in health can be classified into:

Descriptive (Descriptive)

Descriptive Analytics is a description of the current situation and contributes to drawing a picture of past performance, based on historical data and through the use of business information and data mining. The use of this analytical element is the basis on which to build the appropriate approach to achieving the objective [11, 13]. Various techniques are used to perform this level of analysis [25]. Descriptive Analytics is the simplest level of understanding and use. It simply describes data without further analysis, investigation or correlations between variables or information elements, while being completely controlled. Descriptive analyzes operate by categorizing, characterizing, aggregating, and classifying data, which must be converted into valuable information to help health professionals understand and analyze decisions, performance, and outcomes [13].

Diagnostic

The use of historical data provides the main cause of the problem and the diagnosis. The purpose of Diagnostic Analytics is to explain why certain events occurred and what are the factors that triggered them. For example, Diagnostic Analytics is able to understand the reasons behind the frequent re-admissions of US patients, using various methods such as clustering and decision trees [11, 13]. Extensive investigation and directed analysis of existing data using tools such as imaging techniques are needed to discover the boundaries of a problem and help users to understand the nature and impact of the problems. This may include understanding the effect of factors and processes that are inputs to the system on performance. For example, the increased waiting time for the provision of certain healthcare services could attribute many important factors, such as patient, provider, or organization-related factors [24, 32].

Predictive

Predictive Analytics works as a descriptive-analytic since it focuses on the use of information rather than just data. It examines existing interpretations and indicators of the past to predict future performance [24]. It reflects the ability to predict future events while helping to identify trends and identify potential uncertain outcomes. For example, one may be asked to predict whether a patient will experience complications or not. Predictive models are often constructed using machine learning techniques [25]. Predictive Analytics uses huge data sets to improve customer experience, delivering better results than conventional business strategies. They are used to analyze large volumes of data, as well as unstructured data, which produce results, to predict future developments. Predicting future developments, based on available datasets, is a difficult task to pay for information science. Such business intelligence programs help to calculate data flows to a greater extent, including the content of social media, shopping experiences, users' daily activities and surveys [11].

Prescriptive

Prescriptive Analytics takes action on decisions that need to be made on a wide range of feasible alternatives, enabling the decision-makers of an organization not only to look at the consequences and expected outcomes of their decisions, but also to identify emerging and emerging opportunities. [24]. This analytical method automatically synthesizes Big Data and provides guidance on a large number of different possible outcomes prior to actual decision making. The decision-maker can take this information into account and act accordingly. The success of Prescriptive Analytics depends mainly on the adoption of five key parameters: the use of hybrid data, including structured and unstructured data, the integration of prediction and guidance taking into account all possible side effects, the use of adapters as well as the ability to adapt reliable feedback mechanisms [24].

Big Data Analytics has the potential to radically transform existing business and clinical models for smart and effective care delivery [23]. They allow the integration of identifiable health information to allow for secondary uses of the data [52]. Also, by recognizing patterns and deciphering associations, they can facilitate autonomous decision making [33]. In clinical practice, Big Data Analytics can help detect the disease early, accurately predict its course, and detect deviations from the healthy state, present complications, and detect fraud. By providing this information, they help healthcare providers personalize forecasts, provide targeted treatment by taking into account the cost-effectiveness of care, reduce resource wastage, and encourage individual caregivers to maintain their health care [3, 19, 31]. Big Data Analytics provides the opportunity to detect relatively low-frequency events, which can, however, have a significant clinical impact. In addition, the homogenization of clinical data and its effective use support a wide range of applications, such as disease monitoring, clinical decision support systems, tonic management of healthcare, improvement of efficiency and quality of healthcare and cost reduction [3, 7, 34].

Areas, where data analytics are expected to produce the greatest results, include: identifying patients who are most frequent users of health services or at greater risk of adverse outcomes, providing patients with the information needed to obtain documented information decision making and thus better management of their health, easier adoption and monitoring of healthier behaviors, identification of therapies, planning, and processes that do not provide proven benefits or cost too much, reduce re-imports by identifying environmental or lifestyle factors that increase the risk or cause adverse events and tailor treatment plans, promote follow-up applications home health management, population health management by detecting individual needs during emergencies or disasters, and finally gather clinical, financial and operational data for productive and real-time resource utilization analysis [3].

CHALLENGING THE FUTURE

As the BigData challenge mentioned above is how to handle this huge amount of information. In order to be made available to the scientific community, data must be stored in a file format that is easily accessible and easy to read in order to perform effective analysis. In the field of health, another important challenge is the implementation of high-level IT tools, protocols and equipment in the clinical environment. And to achieve this goal, scientists from diverse backgrounds, such as biology, computing, statistics, and mathematics, must work together [3, 10, 25].

Data heterogeneity is another challenge in analyzing big data. The sheer size and extremely heterogeneous nature of Big Data's health make it difficult to draw conclusions when using conventional analysis technologies. The most common platforms for running software that makes Big Data analytics feasible are high computing clusters via computing infrastructure. Cloud computing is such a system since it has virtual storage technologies and provides reliable services. It offers high reliability, scalability, and autonomy along with dynamic resource discovery and availability. Such platforms can act as receivers for the ubiquitous sensors, like computers for analyzing and interpreting data, as well as providing the user with visualized data to make them more understandable.

In addition, in the so-called Internet of Things, Big Data can be processed and analyzed closer to the source of data, using the mobile and cloud computing services. Advanced algorithms are required to implement machine learning and artificial intelligence approaches to analyze Big Data server clusters. A programming language suitable for editing Big Data (eg Python, R or other languages) could be used for writing algorithms or software. Therefore, a good knowledge of biology and IT management of Big Data from biomedical research is required. Among the various platforms used to process Big Data, Hadadoop and Apache Spark are the most widely used [10, 25]. Big Data, and its analysis, make it possible to exploit myriad-like, structured and non-data sources of data, and will undoubtedly play a vital role in the way healthcare is delivered in the future. One can already see a range of analytics capabilities being used, helping to make decisions and improve the performance of healthcare staff and the evolution of the patient's health course. Beyond their significant health benefits, Big Data faces a number of challenges such as privacy, accuracy, and reliability, etc. Further, it should be noted that electronic health data remains largely untapped, and the need to convert processed data into useful and effective information is therefore imperative.

Obviously, the need for further research in the field of homogenization and harmonization of continuous and discrete morphometrical data, there is an equally important need for the development of new processing techniques. Research related to the extraction of biological markers and "poaching" motifs for understanding and predicting disease outbreaks has shown remarkable potential for providing information that can be transposed into action. However, there are opportunities to develop algorithms to deal with data filtering, insertion, transformation, attribute extraction, attribute selection and so on. In addition, with the credibility and improvement of machine learning algorithms, there are opportunities to improve and develop robust CDSSs for clinical prediction, prescription, and diagnosis.

REFERENCES

[1] Garapati, SL; Garapati, S. Application of Big Data Analytics: An Innovation in Health Care. *International Journal of Computational Intelligence Research*, 2018, 14(1), 15-27.

[2] Shafqat, S; Kishwer, S; Rasool, R; Junaid, Q; Tehmina, A; Hafiz, FA. Big Data Analytics enhanced healthcare systems: a review. *J Supercomput*, 2018.

[3] Raghupathi, W; Raghupathi, V. Big Data Analytics in healthcare: promise and potential. *Health Inf Sci Syst.*, 2014, 2, 3. doi:10.1186/2047-2501-2-3.

[4] Ahmad, Z; Tripathi, MM. Approaches of Big Data in Healthcare: A Critical Review. *International Journal of Advanced Research in Computer Science*, 2018, 9(2), 122-127.

[5] Fernandes, L; O'Connor, M; Weaver, V. Big Data, bigger outcomes: Healthcare is embracing the Big Data movement, hoping to revolutionize HIM by distilling vast collection of data for specific analysis. *J AHIMA*, 2012, 83(10), 38-43.

[6] Fernald, GH; Capriotti, E; Daneshjou, R; Karczewski, KJ; Altman, RB. Bioinformatics challenges for personalized medicine. *Bioinformatics*, 2011, 27(13), 1741–1748.

[7] Mehta, N; Pandit, A. Concurrence of Big Data Analytics and healthcare: A systematic review. *International Journal of Medical Informatics*, 2018, 114, 57–65.

[8] Manyika, J; Chui, M; Brown, B; Dobbs, R; Roxburgh, R; et al. Big Data: The Next Frontier for Innovation, Competition, and Productivity. *McKinsey Global Institute.*, 2011.

[9] Belle, A; Thiagarajan, R; Soroushmehr, R; Navidi, F; Beard, D; Najarian, K. Big Data Analytics in Healthcare. *BioMed Research International*, 2015.

[10] Dash, S; Shakyawar, SK; Sharma, M; Kaushik, S. Big Data in healthcare: management, analysis and future prospects. *J Big Data*, 2019, 6, 54.

[11] Sonnati, R. Improving Healthcare Using Big Data Analytics. *International Journal of Scientific & Technology Research*, 2017, 6(03), 142-146.

[12] Borckardt, JJ; Nash, MR; Murphy, MD; Moore, M; Shaw, D; O'Neil, P. Clinical practice as natural laboratory for psychotherapy research: a guide to case-based time-series analysis. *The American Psychologist*, 2018, 63(2), 77-95.

[13] Senthilkumar, SA; Bharatendara, K. Rai, Amruta A Meshram, Angappa Gunasekaran, Chandrakumarmangalam S. *Big Data in Healthcare Management: A Review of Literature. American Journal of Theoretical and Applied Business*, 2018, 4(2), 57-69.

[14] Sarwar, MU; Hanify, MK; Talibz, R; Mobeenx, A; Aslam, M. A Survey of Big Data Analytics in Healthcare. *(IJACSA) International Journal of Advanced Computer Science and Applications*, 2017, 8(6), 355-359.

[15] Institute for Health Technology Transformation. *Transforming Health Care through Big Data Strategies for leveraging Big Data in the health care industry.*, 2013.

[16] Bello-Orgaz, G; Jung, JJ; Camacho, D. Social Big Data: Recent achievements and new challenges. *Inf. Fusion*, 2015, 28, 45-49. doi:10.1016/j. inffus.2015.08.005.

[17] Davenport, TH; Patil, DJ. Data scientist: the sexiest job of the 21st century. *Harvard Business Review*, 2012, 90(10), 70-76.

[18] Huang, BE; Mulyasasmita, W; Rajagopal, G. The path from big data to precision medicine. *Expert Rev. Precis. Med. Drug Dev.*, 2016, 1(3), 129–143.

[19] Auffray, C; Balling, R; Barroso, I; Bencze, L; Benson, M; Bergeron, J; et al. Making sense of big data in health research: towards an EU action plan, *Genome Med.*, 2016, 8.

[20] Rumsfeld, JS; Joynt, KE; Maddox, TM. Big data analytics to improve cardiovascular care: promise and challenges. *Nat. Rev. Cardiol.*, 2016, 13, 350–359.

[21] McAfee, A; Brynjolfsson, E; Davenport, TH; Patil, DJ; Barton, D. Big data: the management revolution. *HarvardBusiness Review*, 2012, 90(10), 60-68.

[22] Fatt, QK; Ramadas, A. The Usefulness and Challenges of Big Data in Healthcare. *Journal of Healthcare Communications*, 2018, 3(2), 21.

[23] Frost & Sulllivan. U.S. Hospital Health Data Analytics Market: Growing EHR Adoption Fuels A New Era in Analytics. 2012.

[24] Khalifa, M. Health Analytics Types, Functions and Levels: A Review of Literature. In *Data, Informatics and Technology: An Inspiration for Improved Healthcare A*. Hasman et al. (Eds.) IOS Press, 2018, 137-140.

[25] El aboudi, N; Benhlima, L. Big Data Management for Healthcare Systems: Architecture, Requirements, and Implementation. *Advances in Bioinformatics*, 2018.

[26] LaValle, S; Lesser, E; Shockley, R; Hopkins, MS; Kruschwitz, N. Big data, analytics and the path from insights to value. *MIT Sloan Management Review*, 2011, 52(2), 21-32.

[27] Ristevski, B; Chen, M. Big Data Analytics in Medicine and Healthcare. *J Integr Bioinform.*, 2018, 15(3), 20170030.

[28] Wu, PY; Cheng, CW; Kaddi, CD; Venugopalan, J; Hoffman, R; Wang, MD. Omic and Electronic Health Record Big Data Analytics for Precision Medicine. *IEEE Trans Biomed Eng*, 2017, 64, 263–73.

[29] Viceconti, M; Hunter, P; Hose, R. Big data, big knowledge: big data for personalized healthcare. *IEEE J Biomed Health Inform*, 2015, 19, 1209–1215.

[30] Chen, H; Chiang, RH; Storey, VC. Business intelligence and analytics: From big data to big impact. *MIS Quarterly*, 2012, *36*(4), 1165-1188.

[31] Bates, DW; Saria, S; Ohno-Machado, L; Shah, A; Escobar, G. Big data in health care: using analytics to identify and manage high-risk and high-cost patients. *Health Affairs*, 2014, 33(7), 1123-1131.

[32] Simpao, AF; Ahumada, LM; Gálvez, JA; Rehman, MA. A review of analytics and clinical informatics in health care. *Journal of medical systems*, 2014, 38(4), 45.

[33] Asante-Korang, A; Jacobs, J. Big Data and paediatric cardiovascular disease in the era of transparency in healthcare. *Cardiology in the Young*, 2016, 26(8), 1597-1602.

[34] Schultz, T. Turning healthcare challenges into big data opportunities: a use-casereview across the pharmaceutical development lifecycle. *Bull. Assoc. Inf. Sci. Technol.*, 2013, 35(5), 34-40.

Biographical Sketch

Dr Andreas Andrikopoulos

Dr Andreas Andrikopoulos elaborated his PhD thesis in School of Medicine, Lab of Medical Physics in Democritus University of Thrace, Greece. His PhD thesis is about restriction of radiofrequency exposure from microwave diathermy units based on distribution simulation upon radiation interactions. From 2014 till now he started to instruct as an Associate Professor at the Department of Optics and Optometry at University of Patras, Greece. He is also employed as a laboratory collaborator of Researching Laboratory of Health Physics & Computational Intelligence (University of Patras) with clinical experience in measurements and prevention issues of electromagnetic radiation since 2008. His research interests include: medical informatics, health-physics, non-ionizing radiation protection, radiation sickness and genetic damage, mechanisms of electromagnetic interaction with living tissue, occupational radiation exposure, electromagnetic hypersensitivity, mobile phone radiation and health risks.

In: Medical Knowledge Extraction … ISBN: 978-1-53617-925-5
Editor: C. M. Koutsojannis

Chapter 3

MEDICAL KNOWLEDGE EXTRACTION: PARTICULAR DIFFICULTIES AND OBLIGATIONS

Constantinos Koutsojannis*
Health Physics & Computational Intelligence Lab,
University of Patras, Patras, Greece

ABSTRACT

In this chapter, the special difficulties of data mining concerning healthcare or medical big data are discussed. Human health care data are the most difficult of all data to collect, deal and analyze. The first important issue is that the mathematical representation and understanding statistical approach in medical data are internally different than those from other data mining activities. As in medicine the primary direction is the care work for a specific patient, and secondarily dealing with him as a research resource; almost the only acceptable reason for collecting medical data is to benefit against the aforementioned individual disease. Software engineers or researchers that are working in other fields will never face the same constraints of primarily privacy-sensitive, greatly

* Corresponding Author's Email: ckoutsog1@gmail.com.

heterogeneous, and massive medical data. The second important issue is the serious ethical and legal aspects of data mining in this field, including data ownership and special data treatment issues. Consequently, researchers should be aware when are dealing with medical databases they may face the possibility that their work will never be accepted or even used from health care professionals if all these obligations will not be correctly addressed from the early beginning. The last important issue is that most of the health care data have particular obligations concerning their openness to other people that are not dealing with the specific patient; their emergency (often dealing with life-and-death); and the ethical commitment to be used only for salutary. Common language, good communication with end-users and mined knowledge supervising only from the field experts, by well-established health care guidelines, are also important aspects that are undetectable issues of an effective data mining engineer. Transparency of medical knowledge extracted from big medical databases is the *holy grail*, resulting in the appropriate acceptance from end-users as medical community members.

Keywords: data mining, medical applications, ethics, legal, expert supervising

INTRODUCTION

"*Data mining*" tools are based on data classification methods in accordance with their final output features, which allow us to discover patterns that we call "*information*" in order to predict future events or discover new "*knowledge*", both resulted from discovered connections between different data "*classes*". To perform data mining, we need the data and the computing algorithms capable to deal with the data. The more organized the data is, the easier it is to extract "*information*" for further analysis using effective tools from other disciplines as Statistics, Artificial Intelligence (A.I.) and Database management (Figure 1). Data mining is commonly used for medical data mining is becoming increasingly essential [1]. All types of data cannot be processed and analyzed using traditional methods because of the complexity and volume of the data.

Data mining provides the methodology and technology for healthcare organizations to:

- *manage healthcare services*
- *improve treatment effectiveness*
- *save and formulate experts' experience that is not included in textbooks yet*
- *provide new directions for basic or clinical research*
- *save or improve the lives of a specific group of patients*

To work with the collected medical data and to extract knowledge hidden under large and different types of numbers, symbols, and words, data mining includes the following steps:

- *Data collection* of a target data set from the original data, on which knowledge extraction has to be performed. This means that a large amount of these contains a lot of "*noise*" that could cover the clear signal that should be uncovered
- *Data cleaning and interpretation* for dealing with missing data, accounting for time-sequence information and interpretation of the reliability of the rest fields
- *Data transformation* using_methods to find invariant aspects of the data coming from individuals' biological and health diversity
- *Data mining* means extracting patterns of important relations by choosing the proper and more efficient algorithms and presents the output appropriately.
- *Data evaluation* by the developer in order to extract knowledge from the mined patterns of established classes (Figure 2).

Data mining "*uses mathematical analysis to derive patterns and trends that exist in data. Typically, these patterns cannot be discovered by traditional data exploration because the relationships are too complex or because there is too much data*". Data mining involves the creation of association rules, the use of support and confidence criteria to locate the most important class relationships within the data. Other healthcare data mining parameters include [1]

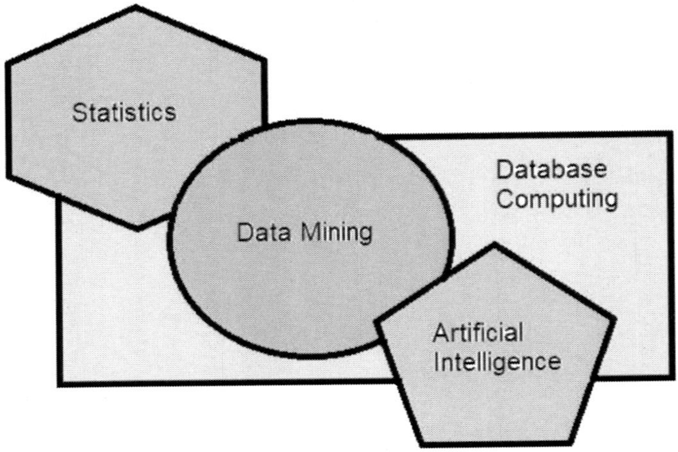

Figure 1. Data Mining is a convergence of many relevant disciplines.

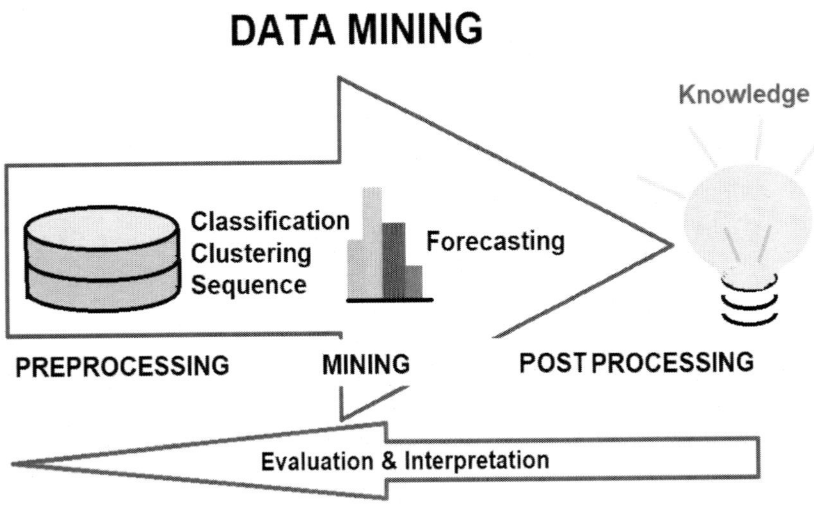

Figure 2. Knowledge discovery from data collectors to new guidelines.

- "*Clustering*" (i.e., grouping a set of objects and aggregating them based on their similarity to each other), or
- "*Classification*" (i.e., looking for new patterns and predicting variables based on the power factors the database contains), and finally

- "*Sequence*" or patterns analysis (i.e., finding paths form one situation to another maybe later, situation), or
- "*Forecasting*", in order to deal with new records that describe usually a new entity, for example, a patient or event (Figure 2).

Usually, mining hospital patient health records, use all data mining techniques including text mining, natural language processing, machine learning, predictive modeling, relationship, and link analysis, statistical analysis, decision trees, etc.

The healthcare organizations as hospitals or governmental health care sectors or even health insurance companies possess rich data sources, such as electronic medical records, administrative reports, and other benchmarking results. Today, data mining in healthcare is used mainly for predicting various diseases, supporting biomedical and clinical diagnosis, advising doctors in making appropriate treatment decisions and avoiding accidental risky events from medical or organizational errors. Additionally, the advantages of data mining are much more than these, as it can provide question-based answers, anomaly-based discoveries, provide more informed decisions, probability measures, predictive modeling, and finally human decision support. Using data mining, healthcare providers can be very effective in such fields as medical research, pharmaceuticals, medical devices, genetics, hospital management, and health care insurance, etc.

Till today because of the restrictions and obligations ruling medical databases, concerning their openness to other people that are not dealing with the specific patient despite the number of publications, there are only a few examples of successful data mining in use in healthcare, but their benefits for healthcare systems are very promising [2, 4, 5, 6, 7, 8]. Consequently, data mining follows a growing interest in the healthcare sector because it offers benefits to care, providers, physicians, patients, healthcare institutions, researchers, and insurers. Healthcare providers and physicians can use data mining to identify effective treatments and best practices as well as to develop new guidelines and standards of care. Even patients, especially those having chronic or high-risk diseases, can receive better, more affordable healthcare services with appropriate identification, tracking and use of appropriate interventions and treatment protocols [7, 9]. Healthcare institutions can use data mining to decrease costs and increase operating efficiency while maintaining high-quality care. This may reflect patient satisfaction and the provision of more patient-centered care. Finally, health insurance organizations can detect medical insurance fraud and abuse through data mining and eventually reduce their financial risk and losses [1, 2].

Dealing with human health care data a software engineer soon realizes that they are the most difficult of all data to collect, deal and analyze. As in medicine the primary direction is the care work for a specific patient, and secondarily dealing with him as a research resource; almost the only acceptable reason for collecting medical data is to benefit against the aforementioned individual disease [3, 4]. Software engineers or researchers that are working in other fields will never face the same constraints of primarily privacy-sensitive, greatly heterogeneous, and massive medical data. The first thing that one should understand is that a diagnostic test that usually provides data for one patient, is one of many values used to characterize the medical condition of a patient; and the final diagnosis is the synthesis of many tests and observations, that describes a pathophysiologic process in this patient, that in western countries should be totally described from the physician. In Western type of medical practicing the doctor or health professional owes to answer to the patient or administration heads, "*why*" and "*when*" at every stage of its' diagnostic and treatment approach and possible answers like "*I don't really know*" or like "*it works, it is OK...*" are not acceptable as in Eastern medical approaches or the so-called "*traditional*". Even A.I. "*black box*" solutions are not permitted from medical community members [10, 11].

MEDICAL STATISTICS AND DATA MINING

The heart of statistical approximation is that the mathematical representation and understanding in medical data are deeply different from other data mining activities because all diagnostic and treatment approaches are imprecise, with serious error risks [11]. The risk here deals with human life and not with money, products, consumer behavior, technical accuracy, etc. Additionally, the variety of biomedical equipment and the aforementioned software cannot easily malfunction or "*reset*". As all experts in biostatistics know statistical approaches are affected not only from the actual data that has been collected but also from "a priori" assumptions of the researchers behind the experimental protocols. The most frequently used statistical tests are designed from the idea of a repeatable experiment, but when employed in medicine this may be subject to ambush [1].

Common problems in medical statistics are [14]:

- *variable classification:* usually undergoes some sort of conversion or analysis following initial collection (real differences or percentage of volume change of a tumor)
- *biases:* when those patients who are lost to follow-up differ in a systematic way to those who did return for assessment, subjects in different arms of the study are treated differently (other than the exposure or intervention)
- *confounding variables:* are those which are linked to the outcome but have not been accounted for in the study protocols
- *standard normal distribution:* that has particular importance in statistics, usually a small number of big deviations result in *leptokurtosis* and large amounts of small deviations result in *platykurtosis*.
- *standard error:* that should be here used to describe the *precision* in the sample parameters
- *tests and p-values:* in order to establish the likelihood that the association we are observing is genuine, or simply due to chance of the selected sample but as normal distribution that in medicine is somehow rare reflects on mathematics of used statistical tests [1, 13] as some statistical tests are designed, not as a search for truth, but as a search for the winning medical scientist. As a federal grant administrator recently observed, many medical researchers who

seek grant funding typically formulate their ideas in terms of "*fairness for me*", rather than "*fairness for competing medical hypotheses.*" [1]

- *the number needed to treat and harm:* the number of patients that would have to receive the intervention in question in order to prevent one adverse event, and the number needed to harm is a similar concept only applied to interventions that have a detrimental effect on patient health.
- *sensitivity, specificity, and predictive values:* Sensitivity and specificity deal with the diagnostic capacity of the test and the predictive values demonstrate how likely it is that an individual does or does not have the disease based on their test results.

The target of the Test	When we use Parametric data	When we use Nonparametric data
Assess the difference between the two groups	*Two-sample t-test*	Wilcoxon rank-sum test Mann-Whitney U test Kendall's S-test
Assess the difference between more than two groups	*One-way analysis of variance (ANOVA)*	Kruskal-Wallis test
Measure the strength of an association between two variables	*Correlation coefficient*	Kendall's tau rank correlation Spearman's rank correlation
Assess the difference between paired observations	*Paired t-test*	Wilcoxon signed-rank test Sign test

Figure 3. Common medical statistical tests.

The usual method in medicine for measuring error *is sensitivity* and *specificity* analysis. Before this one should distinguish between a test and a final diagnosis in medicine because they are different and both tests and diagnoses are subject to sensitivity/specificity analysis [3, 12].

Accuracy calculations are different in medical fields or health care administration. In the end, the most important factor may be the "*false positive*" or "*false negative*" real numbers and not the "*positive predictive*" or "*total accuracy*" values. This happens because dealing with specific patient's life doctors don't care about the "*mean*" but the "*upper or lower limit*" values in order to decide.

All the above limitations of biostatistics, data mining strive toward discovering some structure in data, draws heavily from many other disciplines, most notably machine learning. Data mining differs from statistics in that it must deal with heterogeneous data fields in health records, not just heterogeneous numbers, as is the case of statistics. The best example of heterogeneous data is medical data that, say contains images, signals, clinical information as well as the physician's interpretation written in short plain text. Most successful examples in data mining are due to advances in database technology structure and access, rather than to advances in data mining tools because due to a subset of data is selected from a large database that most data mining tools are actually applied.

As a result, in day-to-day clinical practice, the details of the overall treatment in a given patient may vary slightly because consent and guidance data vary from patient to patient. This is called "*evidence-based*" medical practice. Another peculiarity of the mining of medical data is that the basic data structures of medicine are poorly mathematical or even logical in comparison with many fields of science. Engineers collect data that they can insert into formulas, equations, and models that adequately reflect the relationships between their measures. On the other hand, the conceptual structure of medicine consists of a description of words and images with very few formal limitations in vocabulary, in the composition of images, or in the permissible relationships between basic terms. Parameters used in medicine, such as inflammation or neoplasia, are real to the physician, such as other sciences such as length or strength. However, there is no comparable formal structure in medicine in which a data miner can organize information that can be modeled by pooling, regression models or sequence analysis [1, 12]. In order to defend it, medicine has to deal with too many different anatomical sites and pathologies. So far, the breadth of this conceptual space has been overwhelming. In addition, some suggestions suggest that the logic of medicine is significantly different from the logic of the engineering sciences [3, 13].

Therefore, we theoretically design a clinical study with a specified null hypothesis and a specified sample size and carry out the study until the agreed sample size is reached. A unit may not be interrupted (proven) by a study if a numerical value for statistical significance has been reached until the predetermined sample size is reached. The reason for this is that mathematical thinking explains the experimental results based on the original experimental design and the expectations that this design brings with it, the so-called a priori thinking. The basic assumptions of the statistical test cannot be restored during the examination. The dilemma created by this paradigm is that there may be compelling evidence that a priori assumptions are wrong before a predetermined sample size is reached, and that these wrong assumptions are harmful to patients.

There is an ambush similar to that of data mining tools, such as *artificial neural networks*, where the paradigm of the training/test set exists. If someone has exhausted the network training observations, they can no longer take the test for those observations: they are fraudulent. Instead, we have to use elements from a different set, that is, the amount of data. Unlike animal testing, the problem with medical data is that we can no longer recruit people, repeat the experiment, and create a different training set. You have to make the same observations ethically over and over again.

A new doctrine is emerging, according to which the methods of data processing, in particular statistics, and the underlying assumptions on which these methods are based can differ significantly with regard to medical data. Human medicine is primarily a patient care activity and only serves as a secondary research area. In general, the only justification is to collect medical data or to refuse to collect certain data for the benefit of a single patient. Some patients may agree to participate in research projects that they do not directly benefit from. However, this data collection is usually very small, narrowly focused and is subject to strict legal and ethical scrutiny. Another problem with the paradigm used in artificial neural networks is that they may want to examine the entire data set for reasons other than network training, e.g., In this case, hiding a subset of examples from the training set is self-sufficient. On the other hand, if we look at all cases, we contaminate them a priori reasoning required for the training course - the test [1, 3].

Consequently, a data miner should be aware of the differences between statistics and data mining and their limitations in order to reach the proper conclusion of his /her research approach from the early beginning [15]:

- *Data implementation* is the beginning of data science and covers the entire process of data analysis, *statistics* form the basis and core of the section on data mining algorithms.
- *Data mining is an exploratory analysis process* in which we first examine and collect data and build a model on it that can recognize a pattern and build theories on it to predict future results or solve problems. *Statistics* is a validation process, theories are first created and then validated to test the data sets. Uses only numeric data types for probability and mathematical calculation and prediction.
- *Data execution is an inductive process* and uses an algorithm such as a decision tree, a clustering algorithm to derive a data partition and hypothesize from the data, *statistics* are a deductive process and not predictions for acquisition and verification of knowledge contains hypotheses.
- *Data mining is not a big problem for data acquisition* or acquisition because it is an exploratory data analysis that is mostly a software and calculation process for pattern recognition in large databases, *statistics* are more required for data collection. All data collected can be quantitative or qualitative, primary or secondary data.
- *Data cleanup when retrieving data is the first step*, as it helps understand and correct the quality of the data to get a precise final analysis. During data cleansing, the user has the option of deleting incorrect or incomplete data. After collecting data from various sources, *statistical* methods are used for confirmatory analysis.

- *Data mining deeply digs previously available unknown* but useful information from large databases to help you make critical decisions. A number of methods are used to find patterns and relationships within the available data. This is the convergence of various processes, including statistics, machine learning, database management, artificial intelligence (AI) and data recognition, etc. because *statistics* are an important component of data mining, which provides efficient analysis techniques and tools for processing large amounts of data.

Data Mining	Statistics
Explore and gather data first, builds a model to detect patterns and make assumptions	It provides theories to test using statistical methods
Inductive Process (Generation of new theory from data)	Deductive Process (Does not involve making any predictions)
Data Cleaning is part of data mining.	Clean data before applying the statistical methods.
Needs less user interaction to validate model, easy to automate.	Needs user interaction to validate model, difficult to automate
Suitable for big data sets	Suitable for small data sets
It's an algorithm that learns from data without using any programming rule.	Formalization of relationship in data in the form of the mathematical equation
Use heuristics thinking (rules used to form judgments)	No heuristic thinking
Classification, Clustering, Neural network, Association, Sequence-based analysis, Visualization	Descriptive Statistical, Inferential Statistical
Biological Data Analysis, Medical Applications etc.	Biostatistics, Quality Control, etc.

Figure 4. The differences between Data Mining vs Statistics in health care.

- *Data mining is primarily used for commercial applications* such as financial data analysis, retail, telecommunications, biology, and other scientific discoveries. *Statistics* are used in every data sample to create a range of new information. It describes the character of the data to be analyzed and examines the relationship between them. Uses predictive analytics to run scenarios to determine future actions. On the other hand, statistics breathe in lifeless data.

Some of the popular trends in data mining are application research, visual data mining, biological data mining, online mining, software mining, data distribution, real data mining, and more. *Statistics* help identify new patterns of available unstructured data.

Due to the advent of big data with a large amount and different data speeds, the decision plays an important role in every field and the prediction of the results is crucial for data mining and statistics. *Data mining always uses statistical thinking to access the results.* In the end, different results of a statistical breakdown are not completely random but are limited by the fact that some combinations of health events are normal or rare. Expert doctors usually recognize these events as common or rare, but the exact probabilities are still unknown [15].

Ethical and Legal Issues

Patient-identifiable data refer to any personal data that can be used to identify an individual (eg, name or registry number). This also includes encrypted data if the solution for decryption is still in existence (eg, new National Health Service (NHS) number) [15]. Patient-identifiable data are critical in medical research and required for the developmental stages of disease registers. The problem is that pursuing informed consent for the use of such data is likely to result in a biased sample and is often prohibitively expensive. The issue of data ownership is an open question in the mining of medical data. In legal textbooks, ownership determines who is entitled to sell a property. Because the sale of human data or tissue does not seem to make sense, the issue of data ownership in medicine is similarly confusing. The corpus of human medical data available to obtain data is enormous. Thousands of terabytes are now generated annually in Western countries. However, this information is buried in heterogeneous databases and scattered across the healthcare facility, without the common format or principles of the organization. The issue of ownership of patient information is unresolved and subject to repeated, highly publicized lawsuits and congressional investigations. Many questions are still open [1]:

- *Do individual patients have collected information about themselves?*
- *Do their doctors have information?*
- *Do their insurance providers own the information?*
- *If insurance providers do not have their own insured information, can they refuse to pay for data collection and storage?*
- *If the ability to process and sell human health data is unreliable, then how do we replace the data controllers who organize and mine the data?*
- *Or should this incredibly rich source of potential improvement for humanity remain unchanged?* [18]

In this uncertainty, doctors and other medical data manufacturers understandably hesitate to share their data with data miners.

Data miners could search this data for adverse events. Obvious medical history abnormalities can trigger an examination. In many cases, the occurrence of incorrect practices can be an error in omitting or transferring data and not all bad medical results are necessarily the result of the negligent behavior of the provider.

Another specialty is data protection and security issues. For example, U.S. federal regulations set guidelines for hiding individual patient identifiers. It is not just a possible breach of patient confidentiality with the possibility of a lawsuit and the erosion of the doctor-patient relationship, in which the patient is extremely open to the doctor, expecting that such private information will never be published. According to some guidelines, disguising identifiers must be irreparable. A related data protection problem can be used, for example, to determine important diagnostic information about a patient's data and to treat a patient if he or she can only return and inform the patient of the diagnosis and possible cure. In some cases, this measure cannot be carried out. Another problem is data security when handling data, especially when transferring data (Figure 5).

Only authorized persons should have access to the identifiers before they are hidden. Because electronic data transmission over the Internet is unreliable, identifiers should be carefully hidden, even when being transferred from one unit to another within a healthcare facility.

On the other hand, for example, recent US federal documents have found that there are at least two legitimate research needs to re-identify undefined medical information:

- *to prevent the same patient's records from being accidentally copied from biased research results.*
- *the original (newly identified) medical records may need to be persuaded to verify the accuracy or to obtain additional information about specific patients.*

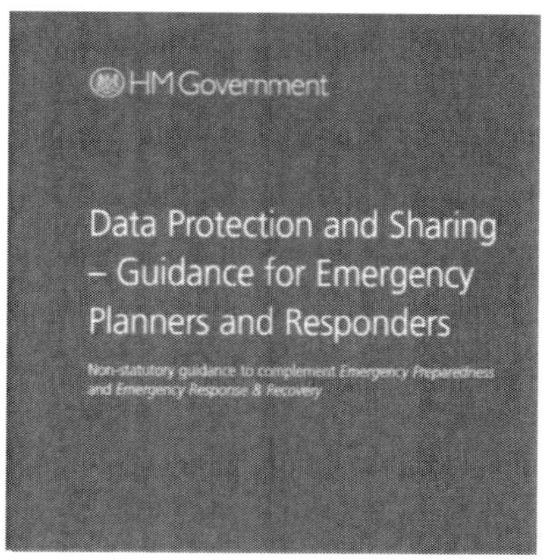

Figure 5. A typical guide for information sharing and ensuring that necessary privacy protection is properly seen as complementary objectives and not competing ones.

These specific requirements could be addressed by the relevant regulatory authorities, but could not be met at all if the data were completely anonymous [1].

Consequently, there must be legal contracts between the organization and all external parties that have access to individually identifiable health information, and must require external parties to protect the information [17]:

- *There must be contingency plans, including a data backup plan and an emergency response plan.*
- *There must be a system for controlling access to information, which includes policies for granting, establishing and modifying access rights to data.*
- *In order to identify potential security breaches, an internal review of data access records must be kept in place.*
- *The organization must provide oversight of personnel performing technical system maintenance activities to maintain access permit records to ensure that operators and maintainers have adequate access, apply personnel safety procedures and train system users.*
- *There must be termination procedures in place when an employee leaves or loses access to data.*
- *There should be security training for all staff, including awareness training for all staff, regular security reminders, educating users on virus protection, educating users about the importance of monitoring login errors, managing passwords, and reporting derogations.*

These and many other rules impose restrictions on medical data providers that would be burdened and inhibited by other academic researchers in scientific research creativity. Researchers need to carefully weigh the perceived need for information that could allow the data to be re-identified in combination with other information [1, 17].

SUPERVISION FROM FIELD EXPERTS

According to the kind of data available and the research question, a scientist will choose to train an algorithm using a specific learning model. There are four approximations:

- *Supervised learning model*, where the algorithm learns on a labeled dataset, providing an answer key that the algorithm can use to evaluate its accuracy on training data (someone is present judging whether you're getting the right answer).

- *An unsupervised learning model* that, provides unlabeled data that the algorithm tries to make sense of by extracting features and patterns on its own.
- *The Semi-supervised learning* that, uses a small amount of labeled data bolstering a larger set of unlabeled data.
- *The Reinforcement learning* finally that, trains an algorithm with a reward system, providing feedback when an artificial intelligence agent performs the best action in a particular situation.

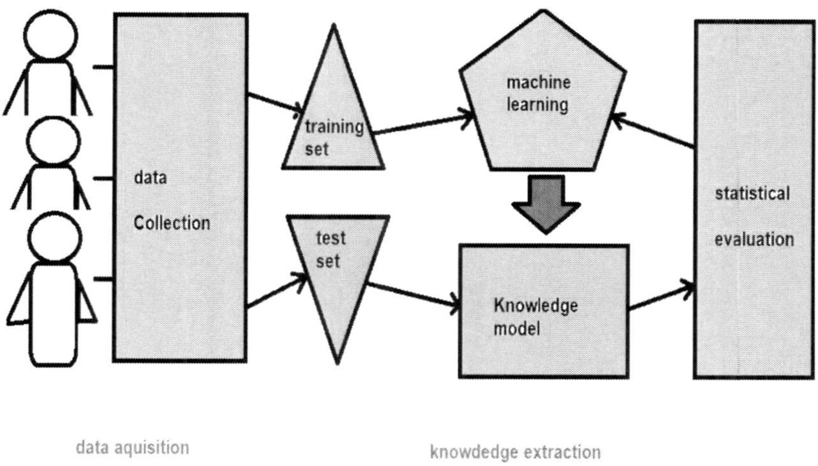

Figure 6. Knowledge extraction from data.

There are two main areas where *supervised learning* is useful: classification problems and regression problems [18].

Classification problems ask the algorithm to predict a discrete value, identifying the input data as a member of a particular class, or group.

On the other hand, regression problems look at continuous data. One use case, linear regression, should sound familiar from algebra class: given a particular x value, what's the expected value of the y variable?

Supervised learning is, thus, best suited to problems where there is a set of available reference points or a ground truth with which to train the algorithm. But those aren't always available.

Clean, perfectly labeled datasets aren't easy to come by. And sometimes, researchers are asking the algorithm questions they don't know the answer to. That's where *unsupervised learning* comes in.

In unsupervised learning, a deep learning model is handed a dataset without explicit instructions on what to do with it. The training dataset is a collection of examples without a specific desired outcome or correct answer. The neural network then attempts to automatically find structure in the data by extracting useful features and analyzing its structure.

Unsupervised learning models automatically extract features and find patterns in the data.

Depending on the problem at hand, the unsupervised learning model can organize the data in different ways.

- ***Clustering:*** That's how the most common application for unsupervised learning, clustering, works: the deep learning model looks for training data that are similar to each other and groups them together.
- ***Anomaly detection:*** Unsupervised learning can be used to flag outliers in a dataset.
- ***Association:*** By looking at a couple of key attributes of a data point, an unsupervised learning model can predict the other attributes with which they're commonly associated.

Because there is no "*ground truth*" element to the data, it's difficult to measure the accuracy of an algorithm trained with unsupervised learning. But there are many research areas where labeled data is elusive, or too expensive, to get. In these cases, giving the deep learning model-free rein to find patterns of its own can produce high-quality results [18]. Maybe the most important issue in medical data mining and new knowledge discovery is that most of the health care data have particular obligations concerning their openness to other people that are not dealing with the specific patient;

their emergency (often dealing with life-and-death); and the ethical commitment to be used only for salutary. A.I. applications usually are not accepted by health professionals. The proper path for effective and usable mining in medicine includes several important steps:

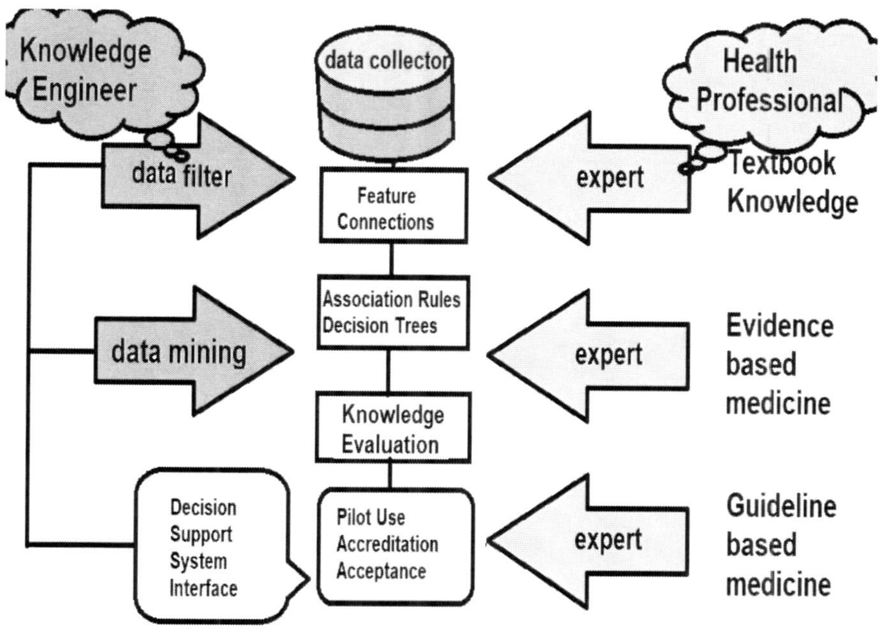

Figure 7. Data Mining and the development of intelligent systems for medical applications.

The first step deals with data, the second with knowledge extraction and the final with acceptance test from the medical community. During previous decades all the procedure of knowledge representation through interviews with field experts has driven most of the promising applications to a "*bottleneck*" or at most to the first pilot intelligent system. Actually, when working with A.I. tools in order to develop a smart system to solve problems or to support human decisions, we describe one that can continually accept, store, evaluate and "*learn*" from new data adapting its' knowledge base after each new entry (Figure 7). Thus the following steps are looping, internally:

1. *Data collection*
2. *Knowledge Extraction*
3. *System acceptance*

One of the best ways to visualize extracted knowledge is through a *decision tree*. Decisions Trees are popular techniques for supervised classification, especially when the results are interpreted by a field expert. Medical doctors can easily accept this type of visualization because it is very close to their diagnostic trees.

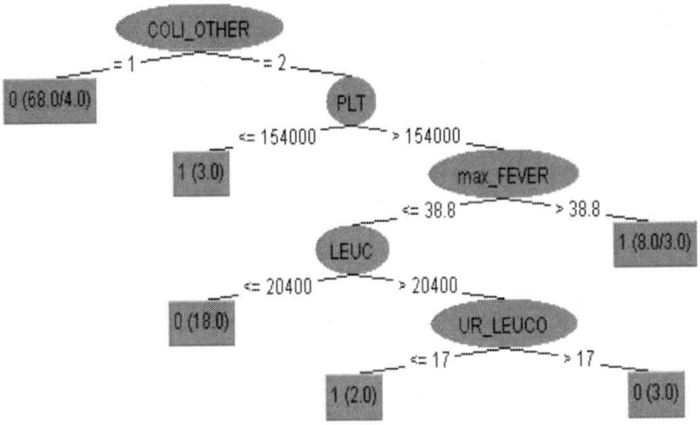

Figure 8. Decision Tree.

The decision tree is a decision support system that uses tree-based decisions and their possible effects, including random event results, resource costs, and benefits. A decision tree or classification tree that learns the value of a dependent attribute (a variable) according to the values of the independent (input) attributes (variables) is used to teach the classification function. This confirms a problem called controlled classification because the number of dependent attributes and classes (values) is given [19]. Decision trees are the most powerful approaches to knowledge discovery and data collection. It involves the technology to examine the vast and complex majority of the data to discover useful patterns (Figure 8). This idea is very important because it enables the modeling and drawing of knowledge from most of the available data. All experts are constantly on the lookout for techniques to make the process more efficient, cost-effective and precise. The decision tree offers many advantages when retrieving data.

Some of them are:

- *It is easy for the end-user to understand.*
- *It processes various input data: nominal, numeric and textual*
- *Ability to process incorrect records or missing values*
- *High performance with little effort* [19]

The tree contains - *root nodes*, *leaf nodes* that represent arbitrary classes and *internal nodes* that represent test conditions that are applied to attributes (Figure 8).

Additionally, it is up to those who create the decision tree because it is not that complicated and easy to understand. Typically, tree complexity can be measured using a metric that includes: total number of nodes, the total number of leaves, tree depth, and number of attributes used in tree construction. The size of the trees must be relatively small, which can be controlled by a technique called pruning [19]. The induction of decision trees is closely related to the induction of rules. Any path that starts from the root of the decision tree and ends at one of its permissions is a rule. These rules can be created very easily.

Common language, good communication with end-users and mined knowledge supervising only from the field experts, by well-established health care guidelines, are also important aspects that are undetectable issues of an effective data mining engineer. Transparency of medical knowledge extracted from big medical databases is the *holy grail*, (as in decision trees) resulting in the appropriate acceptance from end-users as medical community members. Finally, the researcher must be ready even for the unacceptable: there are situations that even the intelligent system has revealed knowledge against national or international guidelines, for example, that uterus cancer is associated most with the number of sex partners or voluntary abortions, or that a group of the supported that entered the hospital during nights or are immigrants will be the most possible patients to die soon in an emergency unit of a hospital and consequently is not helpful for the doctors or other health professionals or counselors that are on the line of guideline-based medicine!

CONCLUSION

According to all previous, human health care data are the most difficult of all data to collect, deal and analyze. The first important issue is that the mathematical representation and understanding statistical approach in medical data are internally different than those from other data mining activities.

As in medicine the primary direction is the care work for a specific patient, and secondarily dealing with him as a research resource; almost the only acceptable reason for collecting medical data is to benefit against the aforementioned individual disease. Software engineers or researchers that are working in other fields will never face the same constraints of primarily privacy-sensitive, greatly heterogeneous, and massive medical data.

The second important issue is the serious ethical and legal aspects of data mining in this field, including data ownership and special data treatment issues. Consequently, researchers should be aware when are dealing with medical databases they may face the possibility that their work will never be accepted or even used from health care professionals if all these obligations will not be correctly addressed from the early beginning.

The last important issue is that most of the health care data have particular obligations concerning their openness to other people that are not dealing with the specific patient; their emergency (often dealing with life-and-death); and the ethical commitment to be used only for salutary. Good communication with end-users and mined knowledge supervising only from the medical field experts, by the well-established health care guidelines, are also important aspects that are undetectable issues of an effective data mining engineer. Finally, only *transparency* of medical knowledge extracted from big medical databases is the most important issue, resulting in the appropriate acceptance from end-users as medical community members.

REFERENCES

[1] Koh, HC; Tan, G. Data mining applications in healthcare, *J Healthc Inf Manag.*, 2005, Spring, 19(2), 64-72.

[2] Mayer-Schönberger, V; Cuckie, K. Big Data*: A Revolution that Will Transform How We Live, Work, and Think*, 2013: Houghton Mifflin Harcourt. Chapter 2.

[3] Moore, GW; Hutchins, GM. Effort and demand logic in medical decision making. *Metamedicine*, 1980, 1, 277–304.

[4] Megalooikonomou, V; et al., Data mining in brain imaging. *Stat Methods Med Res*, 2000, **9**(4), p. 359-94.

[5] Nayak, L; et al., Computational neuroscience and neuroinformatics: Recent progress and resources. *J Biosci*, 2018, **43**(5), p. 1037-1054.

[6] Kourou, K; et al., Machine learning applications in cancer prognosis and prediction. *Comput Struct Biotechnol J*, 2015, **13**, p. 8-17.

[7] Vougas, K; et al., Machine learning and data mining frameworks for predicting drug response in cancer: An overview and a novel in silico screening process based on association rule mining. *Pharmacol Ther*, 2019, p. 107395.

[8] Dimitrov, DV. Medical Internet of Things and Big Data in Healthcare. *Healthc Inform Res*, 2016, **22**(3), p. 156-63.

[9] Ventola, CL. Big Data, and Pharmacovigilance: Data Mining for Adverse Drug Events and Interactions. *PT*, 2018, **43**(6), p. 340-351.

[10] Manning, CD; Schuetze, H. *Foundations of statistical natural language processing*. Cambridge (MA): MIT Press, 2000.

[11] Friston, KJ. *Statistical parametric mapping: the analysis of functional brain images*. 1st ed. 2007, Amsterdam; Boston: Elsevier/Academic Press. 647 p.

[12] Cios, KJ; Moore, GW. *Medical data mining and knowledge discovery: an overview*. In: *Cios KJ, editor. Medical data mining and knowledge discovery*. Heidelberg: Springer, 2000, p. 1–16, [chapter 1].

[13] Brewka, G; Dix, J; Konolige, K. Nonmonotonic reasoning: an overview. *CSLI Lecture Notes*, No. 73, ISBN 1-881526-83-6, 1997, p. 179.

[14] Petrie, A; Sabin, C. *Medical statistics at a glance*. Chichester: John Wiley & Sons Ltd, 2009.

[15] EDUCBA www.educba.com/data-mining-vs-statistics/ (accessed 16 January 2020).

[16] Data Protection and Sharing– Guidance for EmergencyPlanners and Responders, https://assets.publishing.service.gov.uk/government/uploads/system/uploads/attachment_data/file/60970/dataprotection.pdf, (accessed 20 January 2020).

[17] Haynes, LC; Cook, AG; Jones, AM. Legal and ethical considerations in processing patient-identifiable data without patient consent: lessons learned from developing a disease register, *J Med Ethics.*, 2007 May, 33(5), 302–307.

[18] https://blogs.nvidia.com/blog/2018/08/02/supervised-unsupervised-learning/(accessed 26 January 2020).

[19] Bhargava, N; Girja, S; Ritu, B; Manish M. Decision Tree Analysis on J48 Algorithm for Data Mining. (2013), *IJARCSSE*, 3, 6, 114-19.

Biographical Sketch

Constantinos Koutsojannis

Associate Professor, **Constantinos Koutsojannis** is currently Director of Laboratory of Health Physics & Computational Intelligence, in

University of Patras. He is Medical Physicist and expert in Medical Informatics. He is teaching Biophysics, Biostatistics, Research Methodology, Computational Intelligence, Artificial Intelligence and Medical Informatics in several undergraduate and master programs of University of Patras, University of Ioannina and University of Athens. He is involved in a number of Research and Development National and European Projects concerning Artificial Intelligence and serves as a consultant in Artificial Intelligence Working Group as well as full member of Project Committee of European Federation of Medical Physics. His research deals with Biophysics and Medical Applications with Artificial Intelligence on diagnosis, treatment and training using methods of Medical Knowledge representation and extraction from patient data record, medical textbooks and field experts. He has published in a number international journals, conferences and books on the fields of his interest.

In: Medical Knowledge Extraction …
Editor: C. M. Koutsojannis
ISBN: 978-1-53617-925-5

Chapter 4

AN INTELLIGENT SYSTEM FOR HISTOLOGICAL OUTCOME PREDICTION OF PARATHYROID HYPERPLASIA BASED ON CT IMAGING

Kalogeropoulou Christina[1,*], PhD, Zampakis Petros[1], PhD, Tsimara Maria[1], MSc, Hatzilygeroudis Ioannis[2], PhD, Gerasimos Messaris[2,3], PhD and Constantinos Koutsojannis[3], PhD

[1]Department of Radiology, University of Patras, Greece
[2]Computer Engineering and Informatics Department, University of Patras, Greece
[3]Health Physics and Computational Intelligence Lab, TEI of Western Greece, Greece

* Corresponding Author's Email: ckrat@upatras.gr.

ABSTRACT

The development and evaluation of an intelligent prediction system for the identification of parathyroid multi- or single adenomas disease or cancer, based on CT images during preoperative mapping, developed with Machine Learning approaches.

Data from 119 histologically proven PHPT patients referred to our Hospital University Department of Radiology-Computed Tomography, were used on a retrospective chart analysis. Based on simple clinical and CT imaging information and criteria such as CT diagnosis, a location of the enlarged parathyroid gland, density in HU before iv contrast enhancement, the increase of enhancement, dimensions of pathological parathyroid and final histological results, data mining algorithms were constructed.

The final developed computer system based on the Random Tree data mining algorithm predicted the best outcome for all participants emerged surgical intervention and compared to the histological results revealing minimal perfect positive and negative likelihood ratios. The intelligent approach revealed better performance than the commonly used only imaging criteria in predicting the presence of multi-, single adenomas or cancer (ca) disease.

Keywords: parathyroid adenomas, ca, preoperative CT imaging, machine learning

INTRODUCTION

Hyperparathyroidism is a malfunctioning condition of some parathyroid glands that have become overactive elevating the levels of calcium in the blood and causing hypercalcemia [1]. In many instances, a person who has hyperparathyroidism doesn't have any symptoms. A person who has mild hyperparathyroidism may have joint pain, muscle weakness, fatigue, depression, etc. More severe cases of hyperparathyroidism may produce confusion, nausea, and vomiting, etc. Finally, high blood pressure occurs more commonly in people with hyperparathyroidism and may need to be treated whether or not the specific treatment is recommended for hyperparathyroidism. For primary hyperparathyroidism, diagnosis MDCT is clinically used which is a multiphase (4D or 2D) imaging technique, for accurate localization of parathyroid pathologic tissue finally providing the introduction of minimally invasive techniques in most of the cases [1, 2, 3, 10, 17].

Today and according to the existed literature approximately most of the patients with primary hyperparathyroidism, have a single parathyroid adenoma, only 10% have a multiglandular adenomatous disease, and a very small a number of them have parathyroid carcinoma [1, 9]. Clinically used imaging techniques are Computed Tomography (CT), ultrasound, radionuclide scanning and Magnetic Resonance Imaging (MRI) and "4D" or "2D" [9, 17]. Imaging is performed to identify: a) the site of and b) the type of the pathology. This requirement for increasingly more accurate preoperative localization of adenomatous parathyroid tissue has been driven by the recent evolving surgical approach to this disease [14]. Using improved preoperative imaging and having available the intraoperative parathyroid hormone (IOPTH) monitoring, standard cervical (or "*4-gland*") exploration has given way to "*minimally invasive*" parathyroidectomy (DIP) for the treatment of single-gland disease and not only. Otherwise, DIP is more invasive and in any case without any results. The existed imaging techniques that are used nowadays offered great help in preoperative mapping although each one has its limitations. Ultrasonography presents an excellent evaluation of superficial lesions but the small lesions, the ectopic site or postoperative necks are the main limiting factors [1, 5]. Addition of Contrast-Enhanced Ultrasonography (CEUS) presented controversial results [18, 19]. Several studies revealed 99mTc-MIBI-SPECT/CT (MIBI-SPECT/CT) for correctly localizing single parathyroid adenomas in patients with the negative US, although without the appropriate anatomic information plus that sensitivity of the method is still low in case of the multiglandular type of the disease, concurrent thyroid disease or reduced radiotracer retention [1, 15].

C-methionine Positron Emission tomography/computed tomography (Met-PET/CT) is a promising method in patients with the negative US and MIBI-SPECT/CT [20]. Additionally MRI diagnosis depends on the knowledge of the typical morphology and location of the parathyroid glands and common sites of ectopic glands. It seems to be effective in locating remaining abnormal parathyroid tissue [9]. The multiparametric MR perfusion can distinguish parathyroid adenomas from the subjacent thyroid tissue or lymph nodes with very high diagnostic accuracy [21]. CT scan has shown in several studies, superior accuracy and better effectiveness as ultrasonography, scintigraphy or MR imaging is a valuable tool for preoperative planning though the radiation dose remains high, 5.2 mSv in case of 2D CT and 27 mSv of 4D CT [3, 17, 21]. CT examination consists of axial acquisitions, sagittal and coronal reformatted images and the enhancement modification comparing non-contrast images to after contrast enhancement imaging and today demonstrate high diagnostic accuracy for single gland disease and high specificity in multigland disease. Some of the limitations of the method are radiation exposure, the necessity of iodinated contrast media, the technical challenges and the expertise in anatomic knowledge.

To expose the patient to less radiation, in our institution we performed and studied 2D-CT in a cohort of the patients with established primary hyperparathyroidism, to demonstrate the pathology and site of the enlarged parathyroid gland. We concluded that 2D-CT scan offers the same sensitivity, specificity, and accuracy to 4D-CT. A novel positioning mapping was included in our study combined with the parathyroid classification system as follows: a *type A* gland is a "normal" superior gland in proximity to the posterior surface of the thyroid or even compressed within the capsule of the thyroid. A *type B* gland is a superior parathyroid gland fallen posteriorly into the trachea-esophageal groove, in the plane of the superior pole of the thyroid. There is minimal or no contact between the gland and the posterior surface of the thyroid. B+ glands are referred to as those near the carotid bifurcation or mandible. A *type C* gland is a superior gland that has fallen posteriorly into the tracheoesophageal groove and lies at the level of or below the inferior pole of the thyroid, posterior to the RLN. The *type D* gland lies in the mid-region of the posterior surface of the thyroid parenchyma, near the junction of the RLN and the inferior thyroid artery. The *type D* gland may be either a superior or inferior gland, depending on its exact relationship to the nerve. The *type E* gland is an inferior gland close to the inferior pole of the thyroid gland, anterior to the trachea. The *type F* gland is an inferior gland descended into the thyrothymic ligament, superior thymus, "ectopic" or within the mediastinum. Finally, the *type G* gland is a rare intrathyroidal parathyroid gland [5, 15]. As a result, based on several studies, CT scan exhibits the highest sensitivity and specificity rates among the imaging methods for parathyroid glands. However, assisting an automated diagnosis system was thought to increase the likelihood of pathology and the distinction between hyperplasia and simple adenoma.

The purpose of this work is to prove the role of Artificial Intelligence (A.I.) techniques additionally to the traditional MDCT technique in distinguishing mono/multiglandular parathyroid pathology assisting precise preoperative localization of adenomas or hyperplasia.

A.I. is approved as a forceful computational method that may better than statistics describe non-deterministic associations between different parameters in the plethora of medical databases [25, 26]. A.I. has found medical applications as in cancer survival prediction and in some studies has demonstrated greater accuracy over traditional approaches [23, 27]. Machine Learning includes several A.I. approaches, mainly consisted of Data Mining tools, aiming Knowledge extraction from data concerning well-defined instances of a situation. In medicine, medical knowledge extraction is presented as a type of decision tree or production rules [21, 28].

The purpose of this article is to use for the first time, the appropriate approaches of Artificial Intelligence based on the traditional MDCT technique in distinguishing mono from multiglandular parathyroid pathology or cancer cases [12, 14].

Patient and Methods

In the beginning, a retrospective study of 230 patients with biochemically confirmed PHPT, was performed at our university hospital. Each patient has undergone 2D-CT with pre- and postcontrast images preoperatively. The results of the computed tomography imaging were compared with operative and histological data, calculating the sensitivity and specificity of our method. Based on the final results, we developed a novel assistant intelligent automated method to discriminate adenomas and hyperplasia, as an additional tool to preoperative evaluation and improved planning a minimally directed parathyroidectomy.

Patient Population and Data Collection

A group of the population consisted of 31 men and 199 women referred to our University Department of Radiology, a section of Computed Tomography in the period 2010-16, for neck CT scanning to reveal parathyroid pathology and guiding preoperative mapping. The inclusion criteria for pre-operative diagnosis of PHPT based on elevated serum calcium > 10,2 mg/dl and serum PHT > 30 pg/mL. All the patients that have included in our retrospective analysis have finally undergone surgical exploration submitting tissues for the final histological report offering available comparison of results (Table 1). The final cohort consisted of 118 patients with 18 men and 100 women (Figure 1).

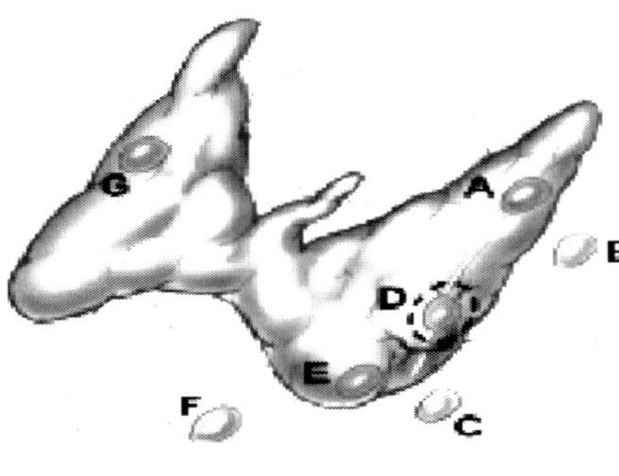

Figure 1. Categorization of the location of parathyroid glands. A: normal superior gland in the proximity of the posterior surface the thyroid. B: superior gland posterior in the tracheoesophageal groove. C: The superior gland is fallen posteriorly and inferior in the tracheoesophageal groove. D: superior or inferior gland in the mid region of the posterior surface of thyroid near the junction of the recurrent laryngeal nerve and inferior thyroid artery. E: normal inferior gland in the proximity of the thyroid. F: inferior gland in the thyrohyoid ligament or superior thymus or the mediastinum. G: intrathyroidal gland.

Table 1. Patient database

18 men	Median age 50 y.o	Older 86 y.o youngest 21 y.o
100 women	Median age 57 y.o	Older 73 y.o youngest 26 y.o
Initial MDCT diagnosis	102 patients with *single-glandular*	16 patients with *multi-glandular*
Histologic Outcome	56 patients with *adenoma*	35 patients with *hyperplasia*
	5 patients with *thyr*	16 patients with *no disease*
	5 patients with *ca*	1 patient with *lemfadenas*

CT imaging was performed with a 16-slice multidetector CT system (GE Lightspeed 16x) and 64-slice multidetector CT system Toshiba-Aquilion Prime). Patients were on a supine position with arms parallel to their bodies. The scanning protocol consisted of two helical scannings: first from the mandible up to the inferior limit of the thyroid gland and the second scan form the mandible up to the superior border of the mediastinum. The parameters for each phase for GE Lightspeed were as follows: detector configuration 16 x 1.25 mm; tube rotation time 0.6s; pitch 0.938; 120 kVp; and automatic tube current modulation. For Toshiba were as follows: detector configuration 80 x 0.5 mm; tube rotation time 0.5s; pitch 0.813; 100 kVp; and automatic tube current modulation. The first scanning phase is performed without *iv* contrast while the second one is carried out, 40 sec after the intravenous contrast injection. For contrast, enhancement was injected 100 ml iodinated contrast material (Ultravist 300, Visipaque 320 mgI/ml) at the rate of 3.5 mL/s followed by a saline flush. Data were stored in PACS. The detailed study included axial plan analysis and multiplanar reconstructions.

In the report was noted mono- or multi-glandular pathology defining the location of pathology using referred classification system [5, 15].

Preoperative Approach and Final Surgical Procedure

Historically the only potential cure for PHPT is parathyroidectomy. The 2013 guidelines for parathyroid surgery recommend that patients with biochemically confirmed PHPT who manifest overt symptoms and signs should undergo surgery [14]. Preoperative preparation consists of physical examination (palpation of thyroid nodules or even parathyroid carcinoma) and biochemical confirmation of PHPT (measurements of the serum calcium, intact PTH, creatinine, and 25-hydroxy-vitamin D). After the decision for surgery, parathyroid localization studies allow the surgeon to attach the lesion by a focused parathyroidectomy for mono-glandular disease or bilateral neck exploration in case of multi-glandular disease (4-gland hyperplasia or double adenoma).

If preoperative imaging studies identify a target enlarged gland, the surgeon resects it with minimal invasive parathyroidectomy (MIP) using intraoperative PTH measurement to confirm adequate resection (biochemical cure is suggested by a drop in PTH > 50% of baseline 10 to 15 minutes after target gland resection). If imaging studies are suggestive for multiglandular disease, is indicated a bilateral neck exploration. Intraoperative PTH measurement is useful for confirming the adequate resection by a PTH drop into 20-30 pg/ml range [14, 15].

Parathyreoidectomies are routinely performed through a 2.5 cm to 3.5 cm abbreviated Kocher incision placed along existing skin creases. Surgical cure after parathyroidectomy is defined as normoacalcemia 6 months after surgery [15].

RESULTS

Data mining techniques were performed using WEKA 3.7.8, an open-source code platform including different AI and statistical approaches [20]. In order to analyze a large amount of the available health records and extract medical knowledge information, a data mining approach is implemented. Data mining techniques were performed using the WEKA 3.7.8 that is an open software source code tool [21]. WEKA is a collection of machine learning algorithms that can either be applied for data set pre-processing classification, regression, clustering, association rules, and visualization or develop new machine learning schemes.

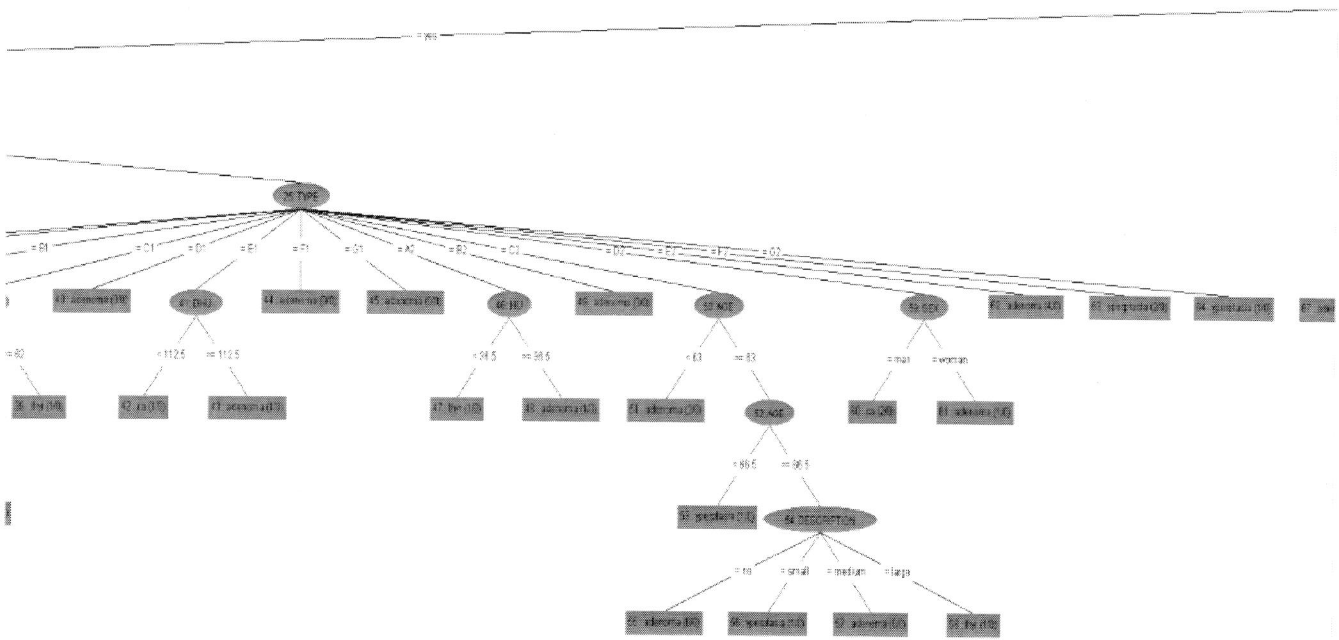

Figure 2. Part of WEKA Decision Tree output.

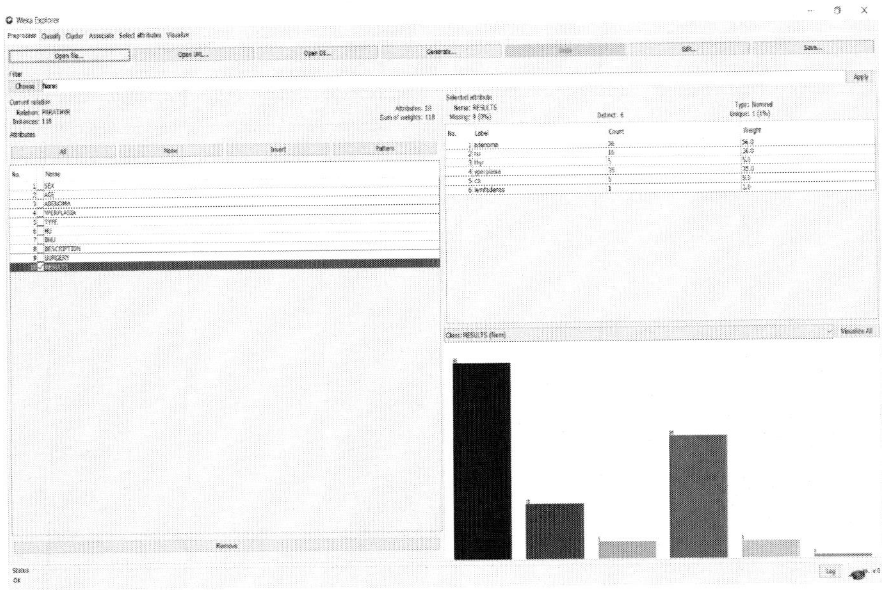

Figure 3. Data presentation.

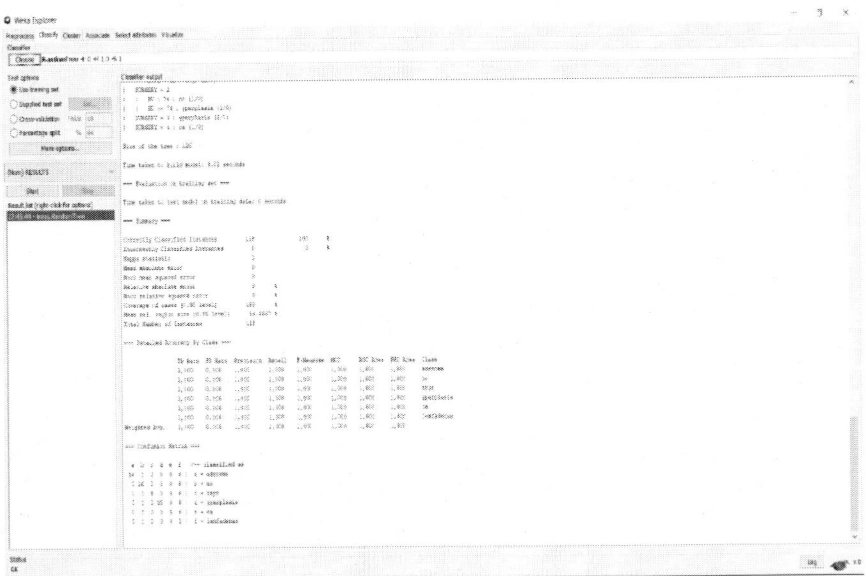

Figure 4. Algorithm classification results.

The WEKA software uses well established mathematical algorithms with a number of the resulting decision trees for data classification [33]. Decision trees can be used either for identifying interesting information or building predictive models as in the present application. A decision tree is a classification tree that functions as a guide to predict based on a series of decisions based on the input data. Specifically, a decision tree is a flowchart (Figure 3, 6) that divides up the data on each branch without losing any of the data (the number of the given total health records remains constant throughout the study) for making a series of decisions. Every time each tree is created as follows: each branch of the graphical representation displays a step where a decision must be made based on the data of an input parameter to proceed to the next branch of the tree. This process is repeated until a leaf provides the predicted output (the type of surgery outcome). As the final step, for each patient microscopically is expected to see a proliferation of a single cell type (chief or oxyphilic cells). Occasionally a mixture of both types of cells can be seen, raising the question of parathyroid hyperplasia. These microscopic features of parathyroid adenoma are challenges for the pathologist to judge each case of being a true adenoma or part of parathyroid hyperplasia [22, 23, 24]. The most important step in this procedure is the choice of the appropriate surgery invasion. Building a decision tree and when it has been grown up to size, an immediate step is required to test the accuracy of the model. From the beginning, the available data were randomly divided into two subsets, a training set that was used to build the decision tree and a test set that was used to evaluate the accuracy of the model. The training set at the present work included 66 percent of the data (78 patients) whereas the remaining randomly divided data were placed in the test set (40 patients). This check is also important since machine learning algorithms present the issue of so-called *overfitting* that is the situation in which the induction algorithm generates a classification tree that perfectly fits the training data but is not generalizing to other instances not present. If we enter the system new data the chosen algorithm continues to develop hypotheses reducing error while the prediction of future unknown values usually becomes worse due to increasing the final test set error [21]. The available methods to avoid overfitting are the pre-pruning and the post-pruning that involves reduction size by removing branches with less power to classify the training set. Pre-pruning stops growing the tree before it perfectly classifies the training set, while post-pruning allows the expanding of the tree to perfectly classify the input set and after cutting branches. The second approach is more effective since it is not easy to precisely estimate at what size will stop evolving the decision tree. The dual goal of pruning is to reduce tree complexity and improve prediction by reduction of overfitting and removal of sections that are based on output error. To create a balance, for one tree to be as simple as possible with as few "branches" and "leaves of decision" while at the same time we will be as accurate as possible ensuring that the produced model will accurately predict a future unknown set of patient data [21, 33].

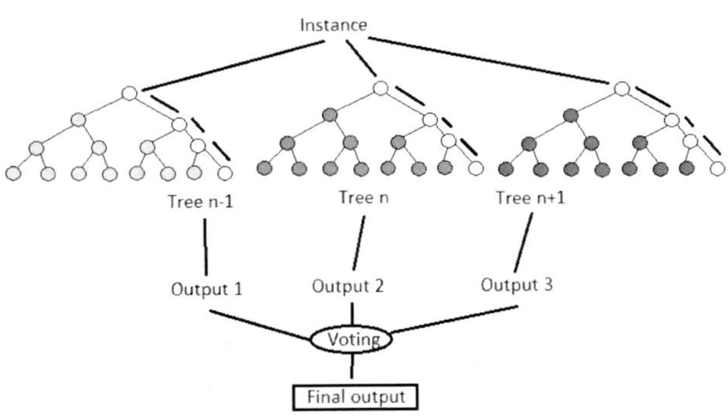

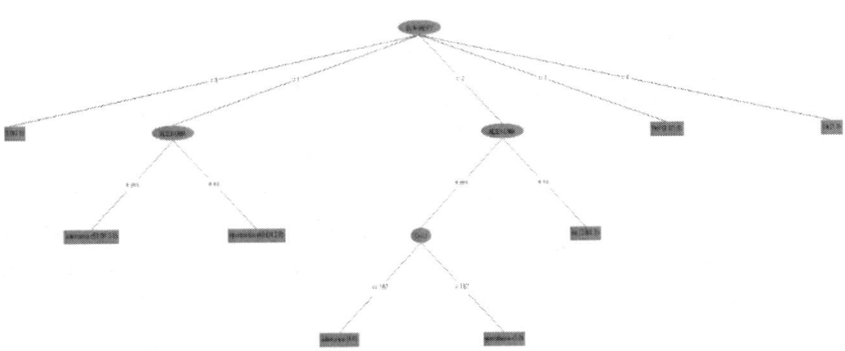

Figure 5. Classification/decision tree for the histologic outcome.

Decision trees are supervised learning algorithms. The main concept, behind decision tree learning, is: *starting from the training data, we build a predictive model that is mapped to a tree structure* [33]. The target is to achieve perfect classification with a minimal number of decisions, although not always possible due to the inconsistencies in training data (Table 3). From the table, we need a decision tree that can be used to predict the type of surgery. A decision tree learning algorithm will return a prediction model (Figure 3). At the start each level splits the data according to different attributes, the non-leaf nodes are represented by attributes/parameters, and the leaf nodes represent the predicted variable or output [33]. The algorithm for learning decision trees follows the steps:

Table 2. Patient database parameters

Input parameters {values}:
SEX with categorical values {man, woman}
AGE with numeric values ranges from ... to ...
ADENOMA with categorical values {yes, no} based on CT image
YPERPLASIA with categorical values {yes, no} based on CT image
TYPE of ... with categorical values {no,A1,B1,C1,D1, E1,F1,G1,A2,B2, C2,D2, E2,F2,G2}
HU with numeric values based on CT image calculations
DHU with numeric values based on CT calculations
DESCRIPTION with categorical values {no, small, medium, large}
SURGERY with categorical values {0, 1, 2, 3, 4} (nr of pathological glands excluded) based on surgery report
Output parameter {values}: RESULTS with categorical values {adenoma, no, thyroid, hyperplasia, ca, lemphadenas} based on histological outcome

starting with the sum of training data

select an attribute or a value that gives "*best*" split

create child nodes

recurse on each child using child data until *all examples have the same class or the amount of data is too small or the tree is too large.*

The main challenge while building the tree is to decide on which attribute to split the data at a certain step to have the "*best*" split. "Entropy" is a measure of the uncertainty contained in a piece of information and is calculated before and after each split. In the training patient dataset, must be selected the parameter that lowers the entropy [33]:

*Entropy = -pP * log2(pP) -pN * log2(pN)*
pP – the proportion of positive (training) examples
pN – the proportion of negative (training) examples

For users that are not familiar with the tool in order to build the decision tree using the WEKA Explorer one can go from the "*Preprocess*" tab to the "*Open file*" button and load the "*database3.arrf*" file (Table 4). Then to the "*Classify*" tab, from the "Classifier" section choose "trees" > "RANDOMFOREST" and pressing *Start*. For the moment, the platform does not allow the visualization of the RANDOMFOREST generated trees. The J48 decision tree is the Weka implementation of the standard C4.5 algorithm which is the successor of ID3. Weka allows the generation of the visual version of the decision tree for the J48 algorithm. So, from the "Classifier" section select "trees" > "RANDOMTREE". Also, the "-C 0.25 -M 1" options are selected for the algorithm with:

- Confidence Factor — The confidence factor used for pruning (smaller values incur more pruning).
- minNumObj — The minimum number of instances per leaf.

Finally pressing "*Start*" the calculation select the result in the left pane, right-click and select the "*Visualize tree*" the final decision tree is created (Figure 6).

SEX, AGE, ADENOMA, HYPERPLASIA, TYPE, DHU, DESCRIPTION, SURGERY_TYPERESULTS

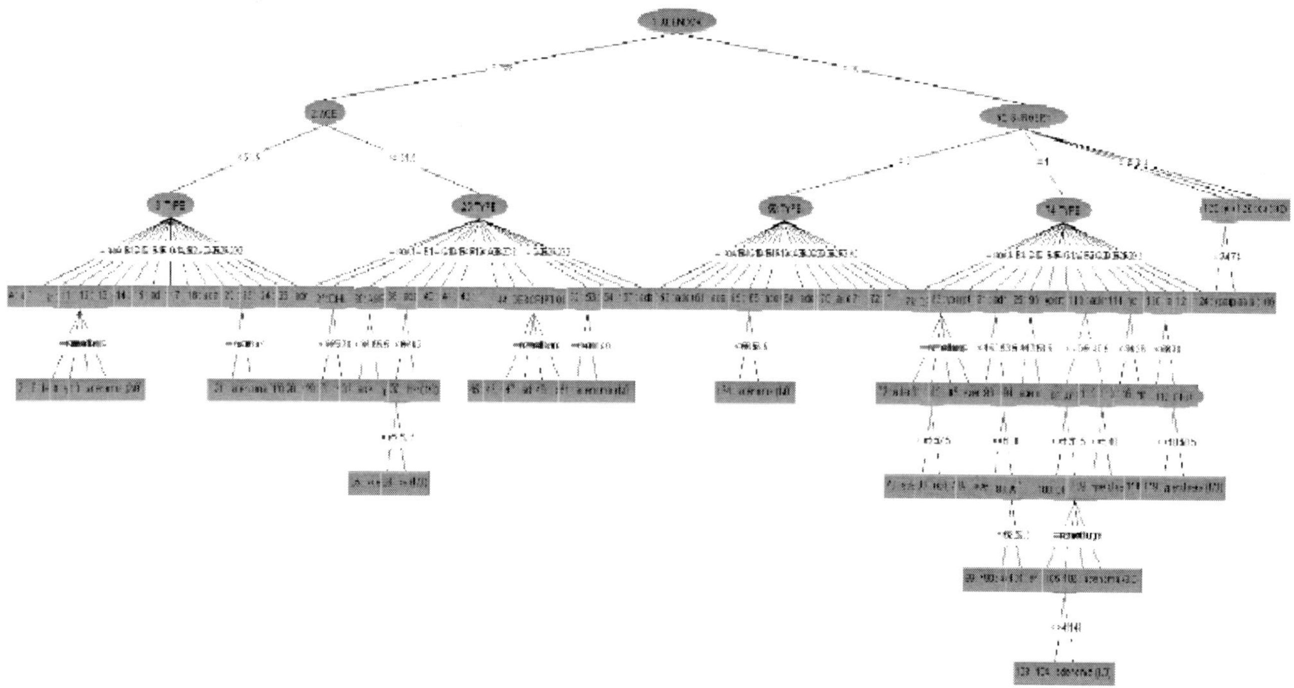

Figure 6. Random Forest Tree. The different colors of the branches represent each of the trees in the forest. The final prediction for a test set is obtained by combining with a majority vote the predictions of all single trees.

Table 3. Part of training data set

woman,53,no,yes,E2,11,103,large,1,adenoma
woman,53,no,yes,F2,40,68,small,0,no
woman,53,no,yes,E1,20,75,medium,0,no
woman,48,yes,no,E2,10,110,medium,1,adenoma
woman,67,yes,no,C2,60,135,large,1,thyr
woman,67,yes,no,C1,60,110,small,2,adenoma
man,55,yes,no,B2,55,175,medium,1,adenoma
woman,72,yes,no,C1,33,157,medium,1,adenoma
woman,59,yes,no,A1,49,184,medium,1,adenoma
woman,58,yes,no,C1,26,202,small,1,adenoma

The Random Forest Algorithm

The final algorithm Random Forest (RF) that has been selected here is a collection or ensemble of Classification and Regression Trees (CART) trained on datasets of the same size as the training set, called *bootstraps* (Figure 6), created from a random resampling on the training patient data set itself [21, 29, 33]. When the tree is constructed, a set of bootstraps, which do not include any particular record from the original dataset is used as test sets while the error rate of the resulted classification of all the test sets is the estimate of the generalization error. Breiman has proved that, for the bagged classifiers, the error is as accurate as using a test set of the same size as the training set [30, 31]. Consequently, using this estimate removes the need for a separate patient data test set. To classify new input data, each CART tree (colored branches in Figure 7) "votes" for one class of output and the "forest" predicts the class that obtains the plurality of all the "votes" [33]. RF has specific rules and is proved robust to overfitting considering more stable in the presence of outliers and very high dimensional parameter spaces than other similar algorithms [30]. The concept of variable importance is an implicit feature selection performed by the RF, and assessed by the *Gini* impurity criterion index [31]. The *Gini* is a measure of prediction power of all variables in classification, based on the principle of impurity reduction it is non-parametric and therefore does not rely on data belonging to a particular type of distribution [32]. For a split (white circles in Figure 6), the *Gini* index of a node *n* is:

$$Gini(n)=1-\sum 2j=1(pj)2$$

where p_j is the relative frequency of class *j* in the node *n*.

For dividing a node in the best way, the improvement in the *Gini* index should be maximized. In other words, a low *Gini* means that a specific predictor feature plays a greater role in classifying the patient data into the two classes. Thus, the *Gini* index can be used to rank the importance of variables for the best classification [21, 33].

```
=== Summary ===

Correctly Classified Instances          118               100      %
Incorrectly Classified Instances          0                 0      %
Kappa statistic                           1
Mean absolute error                       0
Root mean squared error                   0
Relative absolute error                   0      %
Root relative squared error               0      %
Coverage of cases (0.95 level)          100      %
Mean rel. region size (0.95 level)       16.6667 %
Total Number of Instances               118

=== Detailed Accuracy By Class ===

                 TP Rate  FP Rate  Precision  Recall   F-Measure  MCC      ROC Area  PRC Area  Class
                 1,000    0,000    1,000      1,000    1,000      1,000    1,000     1,000     adenoma
                 1,000    0,000    1,000      1,000    1,000      1,000    1,000     1,000     no
                 1,000    0,000    1,000      1,000    1,000      1,000    1,000     1,000     thyr
                 1,000    0,000    1,000      1,000    1,000      1,000    1,000     1,000     yperplasia
                 1,000    0,000    1,000      1,000    1,000      1,000    1,000     1,000     ca
                 1,000    0,000    1,000      1,000    1,000      1,000    1,000     1,000     lemfadenas
Weighted Avg.    1,000    0,000    1,000      1,000    1,000      1,000    1,000     1,000

=== Confusion Matrix ===

  a  b  c  d  e  f   <-- classified as
 56  0  0  0  0  0 |  a = adenoma
  0 16  0  0  0  0 |  b = no
  0  0  5  0  0  0 |  c = thyr
  0  0  0 35  0  0 |  d = yperplasia
  0  0  0  0  5  0 |  e = ca
  0  0  0  0  0  1 |  f = lemfadenas
```

Figure 7. Prognosis classification results with zero FP and only one FN.

We also tested the dataset with alternative knowledge extraction algorithms (as J48, REPTree, RandomTree, RF, LMT) in the form of knowledge decision trees (Figure 7). The following were calculated: sensitivity (the probability that a test will indicate *'surgery_type'* among those with the surgery), specificity (the fraction of those without the disease who will have a negative test result), positive prognostic value and negative prognostic value. Finally, we used the best model according to metrics as sensitivity, specificity and prognostic value [20, 21]. The best results from our experiments were succeeded with RANDOMFOREST algorithm for all different patient groups of *SUREGRY_TYPE* are presented in Table 4.

According to our results, we can see that the trained intelligent system based on training data of patients included in this study has high performance providing no false positive (FP or LR+) results [Figure 8]. This means that for every new patient it can be proposed the proper surgery intervention very accurately with LR- = *0.00* compared with *0.63* that resulted in the traditional approach and perfect sensitivity and specificity (Table 4).

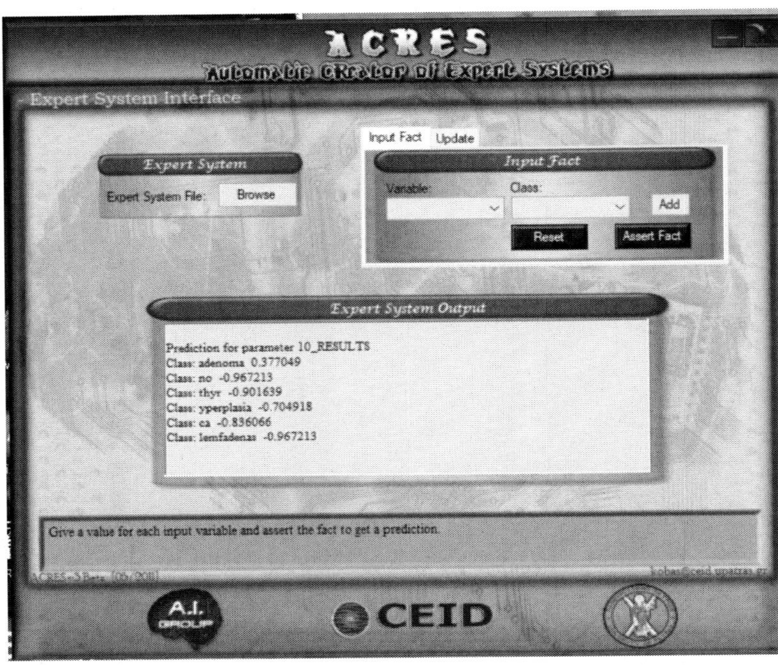

Figure 8. The ACRES v3.0.1 platform for intelligent system creation.

Table 4. Classification results for ca prediction

Input parameters	True positive	True negative	False Positive	False Negative	Sensitivity %	Specificity %	LR -	LR +	Accuracy
Computer System	5	113	0	0	*100,00*	*100,00*	*0,00*	-	*100,00*
Traditional Approach	2	108	3	5	*40,00*	*95,98*	*0,63*	*9.04*	*93.92*

After the final construction of the decision tree, the final model was build up as a computer application with *ACRES v3.0.1* platform that is an ES developing tool (Figure 8). This tool constructs ESs form data and has been developed from the *AI Group* of Computer Engineering Department of the University of Patras [23]. At the end of this procedure, the user can interact with a form that asking for the input parameters of a new patient and giving as an output, using internally the ES, the possible depression type, combined with the appropriate possibility as a percentage. The final tool can be easily downloaded on a mobile system for fast and on-site use by the health professional. At present is used online from mobile phones [23]. In the future and after the collection of a new group of patient records the system can update the internal reasoning model, recalculate its' new performance and give even more accurate results. The internal model could change both with future changes in general knowledge that will be absorbed in newly established questionnaires, or experts' final approach according to their experience [33].

DISCUSSION

AI has proven superiority over linear statistical models in previous reports from the medical field [25, 26]. Experience from the use of A.I. such as its prognostic and diagnostic value in acute pancreatitis and pancreatic cancer showed that the management of these kinds of disorders could be greatly improved from these predictive systems [27, 28]. To elaborate there are many medical applications of for example of Artificial Neural Networks in bibliography including cancer survival prediction, outcome prediction in patients suffering from colorectal, staging and image analysis in non-small lung cell carcinoma and breast cancer [27, 28].

A.I. has been also widely used in the prediction of mortality and treatment outcomes in an elderly population undergoing surgery for hip fractures [28] and age-associated neurological diseases such as Alzheimer disease [28] and other cognitive impairments. Concerning our research, and according to our knowledge this is the first study that evaluates the prognostic value of AI techniques based on CT images for preoperative mapping and offering clinicians useful information for the final histologic outcome or a decision support system to apply minimally invasive excision of parathyroid adenomas.

In our work, we used five data mining algorithms available at the WEKA software tool. Nevertheless, the results of all algorithms were satisfactory, but *RandomForest* algorithm yielded the best results. According to their mathematical approach, it can be explained only from the type and structure of our data [20]. More patient data could result in faster or even different algorithm performances among data mining techniques. Finally, according to our results, we could predict the presence of *ca* with *sensitivity: 100.00%, specificity: 100,00%, LR-: 0,00* with the overall accuracy was at 100,00% (Table 4).

Despite the effectiveness of the above models, there are some limitations [21] that need to be improved to be more accurate as it seems that sometimes the model incorrectly classifies some of the data. This may be attributed to the fact that the choice of an acceptable percentage of errors as the choice between false positive or false negative option depends on the model creator that sometimes cannot distinguish them (Table 3).

This study reveals that the most important application of AI is in extremely complex medical situations where the prognostic factors and their relationships, which might influence the treatment decision, are not detectable in most common statistic algorithms [23, 28]. Software tools as WEKA usually include A.I. as well as statistical approaches that the user could compare to have the best output [27, 33]. According to our study, the surgeon can predict the number of pathologic adenomas using a simple and fast AI system stored in a mobile platform as an IPhone with very good results even if it is controversial to radiologist's results.

CONCLUSION

The decision of minimally invasive parathyroidectomy or extensive bilateral neck exploration depends on preoperative imaging studies.

Adjusting αv application of A.I. in clinical practice can be demonstrated beneficial as it could facilitate health professionals in taking critical and evidence-based medical decisions provided through fast and simply used as mobile applications. At present, the prototype system is used on-line from mobile phones [23]. In the future and after the collection of a new group of patient records the system can update the internal reasoning model, recalculate its' new performance and give even more accurate results [33].

REFERENCES

[1] Douglas Phillips, C., MD, FACR, and Deborah R. Shatzkes, MD, *Imaging of the Parathyroid Glands Semin Ultrasound CT MRI* 33:123-129 © 2012 Elsevier Inc.

[2] Geneva J. Randall, Philip B. Zald, James I. Cohen, Bronwyn E. Hamilton. *Contrast-Enhanced MDCT Characteristics of Parathyroid Adenomas AJR* 2009; 193:W139–W1430361–803X/09/1932–W139.

[3] Chazen, J. L., A. Gupta, A. Dunning, C. D. Phillips. Diagnostic Accuracy of 4D-CT for Parathyroid Adenomas and Hyperplasia. *AJNR Am J Neuroradiol* 33:429 –33 _ Mar 2012.

[4] Jenny K. Hoang, MBBS, Won-kyung Sung, MBBS, Manisha Bahl, MD C. Douglas Phillips, MD How to Perform Parathyroid. 4D CT: Tips and Traps for Technique and Interpretation. *Radiology*: Volume 270: Number 1—January 2014 n radiology.rsna.org.

[5] Steven E. Rodgers, George J. Hunter, Leena M. Hamberg, Dawid Schellingerhout, David B. Doherty, Gregory D. Ayers, Suzanne E. Shapiro, Beth S. Edeiken, Mylene T. Truong, Douglas B. Evans, Jeffrey E. Lee, Nancy D. Perrier. Improved preoperative planning for directed parathyroidectomy with4-dimensional computed tomography. *Surgery* 2006; 140:932-41.

[6] Kelly, H. R., L. M. Hamberg, and G. J. Hunter 4D-CT for Preoperative Localization of Abnormal Parathyroid Glands in Patients with Hyperparathyroidism: Accuracy and Ability to Stratify

Patients by Unilateral versus Bilateral Disease in Surgery-Naive and Re-Exploration Patients. *AJNR Am J Neuroradiol* 35:176–81 Jan 2014.

[7] Timothy A Platz, Moshim Kukar, Rania Elmarzouky, William Cance, Ahmed Abdelhalim Low dose four-dimensional computerized tomography with volume rendering reconstruction for primary hyperparathyroidism: How I do it? *World J Radiol* 2014 September 28; 6(9): 726-729.

[8] David Fustera,d, Jose'-Vicente Torregrosab, Beatriz Domenecha, Oriol Sola` a, Gloria Martı'nc, Joan Casellasc, Xavier Setoaina,d, Africa Muxı'a,d and Francesca Ponsa,d Dual-phase 99mTc-MIBI scintigraphy to assess calcimimetic effect in patients on haemodialysis with secondary hyperparathyroidism.

[9] Nathan A. Johnson, Mitchell E. Tublin, Jennifer B. Ogilvie, Parathyroid Imaging: Technique and Role in the Preoperative Evaluation of Primary Hyperparathyroidism. *AJR* 2007; 88:1706–17150361–803X/07/1886–1706.

[10] Michael D. Beland William W. Mayo-Smith David J. Grand Jason T. Machan Jack M. Monchik Dynamic MDCT for Localization of Occult Parathyroid Adenomas in 26 Patients With Primary *Hyperparathyroidism AJR* 2011; 196:61–65 0361–803X/11/1961–61.

[11] Nancy D. Perrier Z Beth Edeiken Z Rodolfo Nunez Z Isis Gayed Z Camilo Jimenez Z Naifa Busaidy Z Elena Potylchansky Z Spencer Kee Z Thinh Vu A Novel Nomenclature to Classify Parathyroid Adenomas *World J Surg* (2009) 33:412–416.

[12] George J. Hunter, MD, PhD Daniel T. Ginat, MD, MS Hillary R. Kelly, MD Elkan F. Halpern, PhD Leena M. Hamberg, PhD Discriminating Parathyroid Adenoma from Local Mimics by Using Inherent Tissue Attenuation and Vascular Information Obtained with Four- Dimensional CT: Formulation of a Multinomial Logistic Regression Model *Radiology:* Volume 270: Number 1—January 2014.

[13] Jacqueline A. Wieneke Z Alice Smith Parathyroid Adenoma Head and Neck Pathol (2008) 2:305–308.

[14] Glenda G. Callender, MD; and Robert Udelsman, MD, MBA Surgery for Primary Hyperparathyroidism *Cancer* December 1, 2014.

[15] Elizabeth G. Grubbs, Beth S. Edeiken, Maria K. Gule, Brett J. Monroe, Edmund Kim, Thinh Vu, and Nancy D. Perrier. Chapter 2 *Preoperative Parathyroid Imaging for the Endocrine Surgeon. Handbook of Parathyroid Diseases: 19 A Case-Based Practical Guide.*

[16] Manisha Bahl, MD, MPH Ali R. Sepahdari, MD Julie A. Sosa, MD, MA Jenny K. Hoang, MBBS Parathyroid Adenomas and Hyperplasia on Four-dimensional CT Scans: Three Patterns of Enhancement Relative to the Thyroid Gland Justify a Three-Phase Protocol *Radiology* 2015; 000:1–9.

[17] Michael J. Campbell, Paul Sicuro, Adnan Alseidi, C. Craig Blackmore, John A. Ryan Jr. Two-phase (low-dose) computed tomography is as effective as 4D-CT for identifying enlarged parathyroid glands *International Journal of Surgery* 14 (2015) 80-84.

[18] Ayman Agha, Matthias Hornung, Christian Stroszczynski, Hans J. Schlitt and Ernst Michael Jung Highly Efficient Localization of Pathological Glands in Primary Hyperparathyroidism Using Contrast-Enhanced Ultrasonography (CEUS) in Comparison With Conventional Ultrasonography *J Clin Endocrinol Metab*, May 2013, 98(5):2019–2025.

[19] Manjunath Goroshi, Anurag R. Lila, Swati S. Jadhav, Sushil Sonawane, Priya Hira, Shetteppa Goroshi, Mahadev N. Garle, Abhay Dalvi, Pragati Sathe, Tushar R. Bandgar, Nalini S. Shah. Percentage arterial enhancement: An objective index for accurate identification of parathyroid adenoma/hyperplasiain primary hyperparathyroidism *Clinical Endocrinology*. 2017;87:791–798.

[20] WEKA. Application of artificial neural networks to clinical medicine. *Lancet* 1995q346:1135-1138.

[21] WEKA Machine Learning Group at the University of Waikato: http://www.cs.waikato.ac.nz/ml/index.

[22] Elias Karakas, Susanne Kann, Helmut Höffken, Detlef Klaus Bartsch, Ilhan Celik, Christian Görg, Andreas Pfestroff. Does

Contrast-Enhanced Cervical Ultrasonography Improve Preoperative Localization Results in Patients With Sporadic Primary Hyperparathyroidism? *Journal of Clinical Imaging Science* | Vol. 2 | Issue 4 | Oct-Dec 2012.

[23] Christina Lenschow, Peter Gassmann, Christian Wenning, Norbert Senninger, Mario Colombo-Benkmann Preoperative 11C-Methionine PET/CT Enables Focused Parathyroidectomy in MIBI-SPECT Negative Parathyroid Adenoma *World J Surg* (2015) 39:1750–1757.

[24] K. Nael, J. Hur, A. Bauer, R. Khan, A. Sepahdari, R. Inampudi, and M. Guerrero Dynamic 4D MRI for Characterization of Parathyroid Adenomas: *Multiparametric Analysis*. September 10, 2015 as 10.3174/ajnr.A4425.

[25] Marchevsky AM, Patel S, Wiley KJ, et al. Artificial neural networks and logistic regression as tools for prediction of survival in patients with stages I and II non-small cell lung cancer. *Mod Pathol* 1998;11:618-625.

[26] C Koutsojannis, C Lithari, I. Hatzilygeroudis. Managing urinary incontinence through hand-held real-time decision support aid. MEDICON 2010, *IFMBE Proceedings* 29, pp. 913–919, 2010.

[27] Burke HB, Goodman PH, Rosen DB, Henson DE, Weinstein JN, Harrell FE Jr et al. Artificial neural networks improve the accuracy of cancer survival prediction. *Cancer* 1997;79:857-862.

[28] Baxt WG. Application of artificial neural networks to clinical medicine. *Lancet* 1995;346:1135-1138.

[29] Breiman L., Friedman J., Stone C. J., Olshen R. A. (1984). *Classification and Regression Trees*. Boca Raton, FL: CRC Press.

[30] Breiman L. (1996). Bagging predictors. *Mach. Learn.* 24, 123–140. 10.1007.

[31] Ceriani L., Verme P. (2012). The origins of the gini index: extracts from variabilità e mutabilità (1912) by corrado gini. *J. Econ. Inequal.* 10, 421–443. 10.1007.

[32] Strobl C., Boulesteix A. L., Augustin T. (2007). Unbiased split selection for classification trees based on the gini index. *Comput. Stat. Data Anal.* 52, 483–501. 10.1016.

[33] Sarica, A., Cerasa, A., & Quattrone, A. (2017). Random Forest Algorithm for the Classification of Neuroimaging Data in Alzheimer's Disease: A Systematic Review. *Frontiers in Aging Neuroscienc*e, 9, 329.

BIOGRAPHICAL SKETCHES

Dr Christina Kalogeropoulou

Dr Christina Kalogeropoulou is Associate Professor of Radiology at University of Patras (UP) Medical School, Patras, Greece. She is head of the department of Computed Tomography at the University Hospital of Patras. Dr Kalogeropoulou participates in the teaching of Radiology of Medical School students and in the Integrated Teaching Courses of the UP teaching curriculum. She participates in the teaching of Radiology Residents and provides diagnostic work in the Department of Radiology in the UP Hospital, in cross sectional imaging (MDCT, US, MRI). Her research interest focuses on liver diseases (cirrhosis and HCC), on the development and evaluation of protocols of image analysis and computer aided diagnosis systems (CAD) in mammography and chest HRCT and on the implementation of 3D imaging protocols in MDCT [CT-Angiography, CT pyelography]. She has also special interest in imaging of parathyroid glands and the application of Artificial Intelligence for the prediction of treatment results. She has published in a number international journals, conferences and books on the fields of her interest.

Maria Tsimara

Maria Tsimara is a General Radiologist currently working in General Hospital of Patras. She holds a master's degree in Telemedicine from the University of Patras and she PhD candidate in the Department of Medicine of Patras, on a topic related to the application of Artificial Intelligence in clinical diagnosis. She holds a Certificate in Telemedicine and Health

Services from the University of Athens. She is involved in a number of published texts in international medical and computational journals. She was teacher in several undergraduate medical schools and worked in health public and private diagnostic centers.

Dr Gerasimos Messaris

Dr Gerasimos Messaris PhD[2], Messaris Gerasimos, PhD[2] of Medical Physics, UPAT is a physicist with post-graduate studies in medical radiation physics. Currently he is working as a Medical Physics Expert and Radiation Protection Expert in the Medical Physics Department of the University Hospital of Patras, Greece. His research interests focus on digital image quality optimization and he is author/co-author of 18 papers in international journals, 12 international conference papers and 6 international conference abstracts. is currently President of Greek Federation of Medical Physics.

Constantinos Koutsojannis

Constantinos Koutsojannis, Associate Professor, is currently Director of Laboratory of Health Physics & Computational Intelligence, in University of Patras. He is Medical Physicist and expert in Medical Informatics. He is teaching Biophysics, Biostatistics, Research Methodology, Computational Intelligence, Artificial Intelligence and Medical Informatics in several undergraduate and master programs of University of Patras, University of Ioannina and University of Athens. He is involved in a number of Research and Development National and European Projects concerning Artificial Intelligence and serves as a consultant in Artificial Intelligence Working Group as well as full member of Project Committee of European Federation of Medical Physics. His research deals with Biophysics and Medical Applications with Artificial Intelligence on diagnosis, treatment and training using methods of Medical Knowledge representation and extraction from patient data record, medical textbooks and field experts. He has published in a number international journals, conferences and books on the fields of his interest.

Zampakis Petros

Dr Zampakis is Associate Professor of Neuroradiology - Interventional Neuroradiology at University of Patras (UP) Medical School, Patras, Greece. Since 2008, he has officially appointed (by the Ministry of Public Health) as the head person of the Department of Interventional Neuroradiology at the University Hospital of Patras. He teaches Neuroradiology to the Medical students, as well as to post-graduated students in Neuro-Sciences. Regarding his scientific –research work, this is mainly focused on Interventional and Diagnostic Neuroradiology. He has also special interest in the field of Head and Neck radiology. He has published in a number international journals, conferences and books on the fields of his interest.

In: Medical Knowledge Extraction ... ISBN: 978-1-53617-925-5
Editor: C. M. Koutsojannis

Chapter 5

KNOWLEDGE EXTRACTION ALGORITHMS FOR ENDOLEAK PREDICTION INTO THE ABDOMINAL AORTIC ANEURYSM

Maria-Konstantina Chasapi[1], MSc,
Petros Zampakis[2], MD
and Constantinos Koutsojannis,[1] PhD
[1]Laboratory of Health Physics & Computational Intelligence,
University Patras, Patras, Greece
[2]Department of Radiology,
University of Patras, Patras, Greece

ABSTRACT

The development and evaluation of an intelligent prediction system for the evaluation of predisposing and morphological factors in patients with or without endoleak into the abdominal aortic aneurysm sac, based on CTA images during preoperative mapping, developed Machine Learning approaches.

They were used in a retrospective chart analysis, data from proven patients with an abdominal aortic aneurysm, referred to our Hospital University Department of Radiology-Computed Tomography. Based on simple clinical and CTA imaging information and criteria such as the distance of aneurysm sac from renal arteries, aneurysm size, atherosclerotic lesions, aneurysm morphology, lumbar artery size, endoleak, extraction algorithms were constructed.

The final developed computer system based on the Random Tree data mining algorithm predicted the best outcome for all participants undergoing surgical treatment and compared with the histological results.

The smart approach revealed better performance than commonly used imaging criteria for predicting endoleak into the abdominal aortic aneurysm.

Keywords: abdominal aortic aneurysm, CTA imaging, endoleak, Random Tree, artificial intelligence, machine learning, knowledge extraction

INTRODUCTION

The Abdominal Aortic Aneurysm

Abdominal Aortic Aneurysm: Aneurysm, we call the increase in the size of an artery over 50% of its normal size. The abdominal aortic aneurysm is an enlargement created in a weakened area of the aorta in the abdomen [2].

Abdominal aortic aneurysms are divided into 3 categories: the adrenal glands, which comprise the abdominal aorta more central to the renal artery, the adrenal glands, which comprise the abdominal aortic aneurysms, which include the renal arteries, and the adrenal glands, which are located in the abdominal aorta of the peripheral renal artery [4, 6, 7].

The creation of an abdominal aortic aneurysm is in most cases a degenerative process. Structural and hemodynamic conditions unique to the subcortical aorta may explain the "preference" of creating an abdominal aortic aneurysm in this anatomical region [2]. The rates of abdominal aortic aneurysms are more common in patients with atherosclerosis, with a prevalence of approximately 5% in patients with coronary heart disease and approximately 10% in patients with atherosclerosis. Hypertension, a positive family history, smoking are potential contributors that significantly increase the risk of the abdominal aortic aneurysm [4, 5, 6, 7].

Monitoring and diagnosis are usually achieved using imaging methods. One way to diagnose the presence of an abdominal aortic aneurysm is by simple abdominal ultrasound (USG).

It is a non-invasive examination that is highly reliable in experienced hands. It has a high sensitivity of 95% to 100% and a specificity of almost 100%.

Axial angiography (CTA) is the dominant diagnostic test providing most information on the existence of the aneurysm and its anatomical features. It evaluates the shape of the aneurysm with more detailed anatomical details of the mesenteric and lacrimal arteries and also provides a better representation of the adrenal aneurysms. It is useful information for planning invasive treatment. It is the method of choice before surgery or intra-abdominal surgery: it is necessary to adapt stent-grafts to cases where endovascular treatment is indicated as it allows the measurement of necessary anatomical data ("sizing") [2] and indicates the existence of a thrombus and the relationship of aneurysms other organs. It uses iodine-rich infusion material, contrast material, and CT scanning to help diagnose and evaluate aneurysms. It is performed on a multi-axial CT scan that uses X-rays to obtain multiple axial images, which are then reconstructed from a computer to provide 2D or 3D images. It has 99% sensitivity, 95.2% specificity, and 98.3% success [7]. In addition, the CTA is the test of choice in evaluating aneurysm before and after intravascular stenting, due to the intracellular calcium detection capability. Another benefit of the CTA is that it allows for a better assessment of blood vessel dilation and can better detect blood clots. In the case where an intravitreal implant is inserted in a patient with an abdominal aortic aneurysm, a post-operative lifetime examination with periodic examination with axial angiography is required to confirm that it is still functioning well and that the implant remains in the correct position.

As a result, on the basis of several studies, computed tomography has the highest rates of sensitivity and specificity among imaging methods [7]. However, assisting in an automated diagnostic system is believed to increase the likelihood of pathology and to separate patients who may or may not have an intra-operative diagnosis.

The purpose of this work is to demonstrate the role of Artificial Intelligence (AI) techniques in conjunction with the traditional CTA technique for predicting endoleak into the abdominal aortic aneurysm sac.

Al. has been adopted as a robust computational method that can better describe statistics than non-deterministic correlations between different parameters in the plethora of medical databases [20, 21].

Al. has found medical applications such as cancer survivor prediction.

Furthermore, endoleak has proven more accurate than traditional approaches [22]. Machine Learning includes a number of A.I. approaches, mainly based on data mining tools, with the aim of extracting knowledge from data on well-defined instances of a situation. In medicine, the extraction of medical knowledge is presented as a type of decision tree or production rules [19, 23].

The purpose of this research is to use for the first time the appropriate approaches of Artificial Intelligence based on the traditional CTA technique for predicting endoleak into the abdominal aortic aneurysm sac.

PATIENTS AND METHODS

The Patient Population and Data Collection

A population group of 42 men reported to the University of Radiology, Department of Computed Tomography, 2013-18, for a CTA scan to reveal abdominal aortic aneurysm pathology and to guide preoperative mapping.

CT imaging was performed with a 16-slice multi-sensor CT CT system (GE Lightspeed 16x) and 64-slide multidetector CT system Toshiba-Aquilion Prime. Patients were on supine with their hands parallel to their bodies. The parameters for each phase for GE Lightspeed were as follows: detector configuration 16x1.25mm; tube rotation time 0.6s; pitch 0.938; 120kVp; and automatic tube current modulation. For Toshiba were as follows: detector configuration 80X0.5mm; tube rotation time 0.5s; pitch

0.813; 100kVp; and automatic tube current modulation. Data were stored in PACS. The detailed study included axial plan analysis and multiplanar reconstructions.

Preoperative approach and final surgery

Indications for the treatment of an aortic aneurysm are:

1. Anchor diameter > 50 mm
2. Anatomical diameter > 45 mm showing a rapid increase
3. the presence of symptoms such as pain, infection, embolism or rupture.

We know from the literature that the possible remedies for treating an abdominal aortic aneurysm are:

1. *Open surgical repair* of an abdominal aortic aneurysm involves an incision of the abdomen and if necessary two smaller ones in the groin areas to directly visualize the aortic aneurysm [8, 9, 10]. The procedure is performed in an operating room under general anesthesia. The surgeon will make an incision in the abdomen either lengthwise from below the breastbone to just below the navel or across the abdomen and down the center. Once the abdomen is opened, the aneurysm will be repaired by the use of a long cylinder-like tube called a graft. The graft is made of very strong durable plastic material, either Dacron (polyester) or PTFE (polytetrafluorethylene) in the size of normal aorta and is either straight or bifurcated. The graft is sutured to the aorta connecting one end of the aorta at the site of the aneurysm to the other end of the aorta. Open repair remains the standard procedure for an abdominal aortic aneurysm repair. The wounds will be closed either with nylon stitches or metal clips, which will be removed in 10-12 days or with absorbable sutures. The graft lasts for a lifetime and is very unlikely to require replacement. The operation is successful in 95-98% of cases.

2. *Endovascular aneurysm repair (EVAR).*The procedure is carried out in a sterile environment under fluoroscopic guidance. It is usually carried

out by a vascular surgeon, interventional radiologist or cardiac surgeon, and occasionally, general surgeon or interventional cardiologist.The procedure can be performed under general, regional (spinal or epidural) or even local anesthesia [11, 12]. Abdominal aortic aneurysm repair is a procedure used to treat an aneurysm (abnormal enlargement) of the abdominal aorta. Repair of an abdominal aortic aneurysm may be performed surgically through an open incision or in a minimally invasive procedure called endovascular aneurysm repair (EVAR). Access to the patient's femoral arteries can be with surgical incisions or percutaneously in the groin on both sides. Vascular sheaths are introduced into the patient's femoral arteries, through which guidewires, catheters and the endograft are passed. In the EVAR procedure, a stent graft (a fabric tube supported by metal wire stents that reinforces the weak spot in the aorta) is inserted into the aneurysm through small incisions in the groin [11, 12]. Endovascular repair of aneurysms does not require a large incision and has a substantially shorter recovery than the conventional open surgical approach. However, not all aneurysms are suitable for endovascular repair.

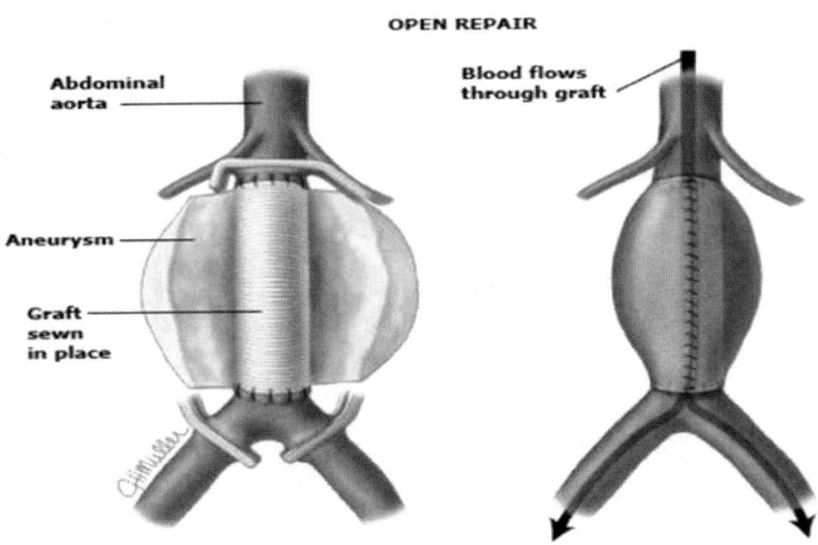

Figure 1. AAA Open Surgical Repair (modified image from [29]).

The surgeon first inserts a catheter into an artery in the groin (upper thigh) and threads it to the aneurysm. Then, diagnostic angiography images are captured of the aorta to determine the location of the patient's renal arteries, so the stent-graft can be deployed without blocking these. The surgeon threads the graft (also called a stent graft) into the aorta to the aneurysm. The graft is then expanded inside the aorta and fastened in place to form a stable channel for blood flow. The graft reinforces the weakened section of the aorta to prevent the aneurysm from rupturing. Specifically, the endograft acts as an artificial lumen for blood to flow through, protecting the surrounding aneurysm sac. This reduces the pressure in the aneurysm, which itself will usually thrombose and shrink in size over time [12].

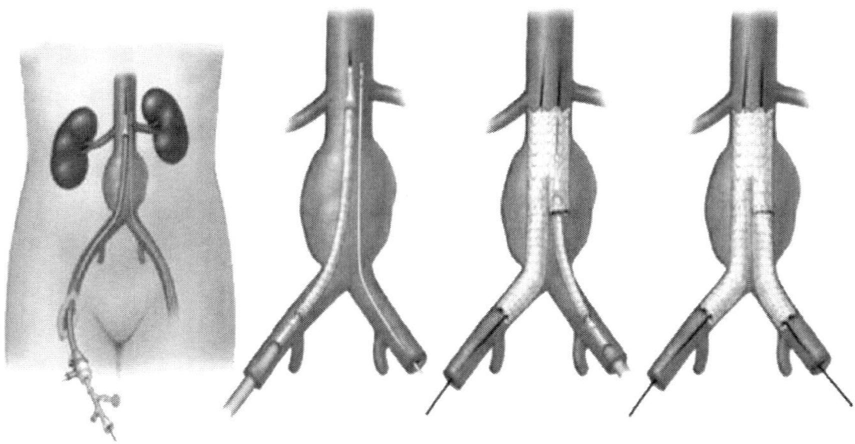

Figure 2. AAA Endovascular Repair [modified image 30].

WEKA Open Source

The Waikato Environment for Knowledge Analysis (WEKA), is a popular software suite of machine learning written in Java, developed at the University of Waikato in New Zealand [17]. It is free software under the GNU General Public License. WEKA 3.7.8 is a suite, which contains a collection of visualization tools and algorithms for data analysis and predictive modeling, along with graphical user interfaces for easy access to these functions.

It contains data pre-processing capabilities in C and a Make file-based system for implementing machine learning experiments. It incorporates different AI methods and statistical approaches [18]. WEKA supports several key data mining processes, in particular: data pre-processing, grouping, sorting, regression, clustering, visualization, and selection of rules. All WEKA techniques are based on the assumption that data is available as a single file or correlation, where each data point is described by a fixed number of attributes (normal, numerical, or nominal, but some other attributes are also supported).

WEKA software uses standard mathematical algorithms with many of them resulting in decision trees for data classification [17]. With Decision trees, interesting information can identify, and predictive models can be constructed. A decision tree is a flowchart that divides the data into each branch without losing any of the data to make a series of decisions. It is a sorting tree that acts as a guide to make a prediction based on a series of decisions based on input data. The process of creating the tree is as follows: each branch of the graph represents a step where one must make a decision based on the input of one input parameter to move to the next branch of the tree. This procedure is repeated until the sheet provides the predicted yield (the intercept prediction). The most important step in this procedure is the provision of an intra-ablation in the abdominal aortic aneurysm.

Creating a decision tree requires an immediate step to check the accuracy of the model. From the outset, the available data were randomly divided into two subsets, a set of training used to construct the decision tree and a set of tests used to evaluate the accuracy of the model.

The training set in this project comprised 66 percent of the data while the remaining randomly divided data were placed in the test set. This control is also important since machine learning algorithms address the issue of the so-called hyperlink, that is, the state in which the induction algorithm produces a classification tree that fits perfectly with the training data, but does not generalize to other cases that do not exist. If we enter new data into the system, the selected algorithm continues to develop error-reducing assumptions, while predicting future unknown values usually gets worse due to the increase in the final set of error tests. The available methods of avoiding placement are pre-pruning and post-pruning which entail the reduction in size by removing branches with less force to classify the training set. Pre-pruning stops growing the tree before the training set is perfectly sized, while post-pruning allows the tree to expand to fit the input set perfectly after the branches are cut. The second approach is more effective, as it is not easy to estimate precisely to what extent the decision tree will stop evolving. The dual objective of the industry is to reduce the complexity of trees and improve forecasting by reducing overload and removing parts based on output error. To create a balance, for a tree to be as simple as possible, with minimal "branches" and "decision sheets" while at the same time being as precise as possible ensuring that the model produced accurately predicts the future unknown patient data set.

Decision trees are supervisory learning algorithms. The basic idea behind learning decision trees is: Starting with the training data, we create a model template that is mapped to a tree structure [28]. The objective is to achieve a perfect classification with a minimum number of decisions, though not always possible due to inconsistencies in training data. From the table, we need a decision tree that can be used to predict escape. A decision tree learning algorithm will return a prediction model. In the beginning, each layer separates the data according to different characteristics, non-leaf nodes are represented by features/parameters, and leaf nodes represent the predicted variable or output. The algorithm for learning decision trees follows these steps:

- starting from the sums of training data

Select an attribute or value that gives the "best" partition. "Entropy" is a measure of the uncertainty contained in the information and calculated before and after each split. In the patient education dataset, the parameter that reduces entropy should be selected [28]:

- *Entropy = -pP * log2(pP) -pN * log2(pN)*
- *pP – the proportion of positive (training) examples*
- *pN – the proportion of negative (training) examples*

For users who are not familiar with the tool to build the decision tree using WEKA Explorer, you can go from the "Preprocess" tab to the "Open File" button and download the "dataset.arrf" file. Then, on the "Sort" tab, from the "Classifier" section, select "trees" > "RANDOMFOREST" and click Start. At this time, the platform does not allow the display of trees produced by RANDOMFOREST. The J48 decision tree is the Weka implementation of the standard C4.5 algorithm, which is the successor of ID3. Weka allows the creation of the visual version of the decision tree for the J48 algorithm. So, from the "Classifier" section select "trees"> "RANDOMTREE". Also, the options "-0.25-M1" are selected for the algorithm with:

- confidenceFactor - The confidence factor used for pruning (lower values suffer more than pruning).
- minNumObj - The minimum number of cases per sheet.

Finally, by pressing the "Start" button, the calculation will select the result in the left pane, right-click, and by selecting "Tree Vision" the final decision tree is created.

The Random Forest Algorithm

The Random Forest (RF) algorithm is a collection or set of sorting and regression trees (CARTs) trained in data sets of the same size as the training set called bootstraps, created by random sampling of compiled data to compile data. of patients. When the tree is constructed, a set bootstrap is used, which does not include any specific record from the original dataset, as the error rate of the classification of the results of all test sets is the estimation of the generalization error. Breiman has shown that, for sachet classifiers, the error is accurate as it uses a test set of the same size as the training set [25, 26]. Therefore, the use of this assessment removes the need for a separate patient data set. To classify the new input data, each individual CART tree "votes" for an output class, and the "forest" predicts the class that obtains the majority of all "votes" [28]. RF has specific rules and has proven to be over-powered by assuming a more stable presence of deformers and spaces too large than other similar algorithms [25]. The concept of variable importance is a tacit selection of features performed by RF and evaluated by the Gini impurity criteria index [26]. Gini is a measure of the predictive power of all variables in the classification, based on the principle of reducing impurities is non-parametric and therefore not based on data belonging to a particular type of distribution [27]. For a partition (white circles in Figure 6), the Gini index of a node is:

$$Gini(n)=1-\sum 2j=1(pj)2$$

where pj is the relative frequency of the class j at node n.

To divide a node in the best way, the Gini index should be maximized. In other words, a low Gini means that a particular prediction feature plays a greater role in classifying patient data into two categories. Thus, the Gini index can be used to classify the importance of variables for better classification [19, 28].

The Random Tree Algorithm

The Random Tree algorithm has been introduced by Leo Breiman and Adele Cutler. The algorithm can handle both classification and regression problems. Random Trees is a collection of forecasts called forest trees, more about what we learn from L. Breiman.

The classification works as follows: the random tree classifier takes the input feature vector, classifies it with each tree in the forest, and extracts the class label that received the majority of the "votes". In the case of regression, the classifier response is the average of the responses over all the trees in the forest.

All trees are trained with the same parameters but with different training sets. These sets are generated from the initial training set using the bootstrap procedure: for each training set, you randomly select the same number of vectors as in the original set. The vectors are chosen by replacement. That is, some operators will appear more than once, and some will be absent. At each node of each trained tree, not all variables are used to find the best split, but a random subset of them. Each node produces a new subset. However, its size is fixed for all the nodes and all the trees. It is a training parameter set to be by default. None of the build trees are pruned. In Random Trees there is no need for any accuracy estimation procedures, such as cross-validation or bootstrap, or a separate test set to get an estimate of the training error. The error is estimated internally during the training. When the training set for the current tree is drawn by sampling with replacement, some vectors are left out (so-called oob (out-of-bag) data). The size of the oob data is about N / 3. The classification error is estimated by using this oob-data as follows [13, 14, 15, 16]:

1. Get a prediction for each vector, which is oob relative to the i-th tree, using the very i-th tree.
2. After all the trees that have been trained, for each vector that has ever been oob, find the class winner for it (the class that got the majority of votes in the trees where the vector was oob) and compare it with the ground -truth response.
3. Compute the classification error estimated as a ratio of the number of misclassified oob vectors to all the vectors in the original data. In the case of regression, the oob error is computed as the squared error for oob vectors difference divided by the total number of vectors.

Progressive Method

The procedure followed in our case is as follows:

We first loaded the data from the .arff patient file, tested the dataset with alternative knowledge extraction algorithms (such as J48, REPTree, RandomTree, RF, LMT) in the form of knowledge trees. The following were calculated: sensitivity, specificity, positive prognosis and negative predictive value [17, 18, 19]. Finally, we used the best model according to the measurements as sensitivity, specificity and predictive value. The best results from our experiments were obtained with the RANDOMTREE algorithm for all patients in the dataset.

To further improve the specific results, we obtained from RANDOMTREE we split our data manually, we created 3 different training sets and test sets to use, the combination of which yields a better accuracy rate and a better decision tree.

Analytically, from the original set of data, by excluding the appearance of intra-escape or not, we separated the data, in patients who showed intra-escape and in patients who did not. Then, out of the total number of patients undergoing intra-ablation, by doing the operation (0.66 * the number of intra-ablation lines), we calculated 66% which was part of the 1st training set, with the remaining lines in the data set, ie the remaining 34% was part of the first set of tests. Correspondingly, out of the total number of patients who did not have an intra-escape, by doing the operation (0.66 * the number of intra-escape lines) we calculated 66% who completed the 1st set of training while the remaining lines of the data set, that is, the rest 34% completed the 1st set of tests.

Having the data of the 1st training set and 1st test set, the next 2 training sets and test sets came up, which we then checked.

To create them, we went first to the first set of training. In a new column of the excel file, we typed = Rand (), by pressing enter a decimal number appeared. We continued this process for the whole number of registrations and then customized the rank based on the column we created, from smallest to largest. This is how the 2nd training set file was created.

In order to create the 2nd test set file, we followed the same procedure. Specifically, in a new column of the excel file, we typed = Rand (), by pressing enter a decimal number appeared. We included the whole number of entries in this process, and then we sorted through the column we created, from smallest to largest. This created the 2nd test set file.

Starting with the 2nd training set and 2nd test set, we also created the last, 3rd training set and 3rd set of tests. In detail, in a new column of the excel file, we typed = Rand (), by pressing enter a decimal number appeared. We continued this process for the whole number of registrations and then customized the rank based on the column we created, from smallest to largest. This is how the 3rd training set file was created.

For the 3rd set of tests, we followed the same procedure. Specifically, in a new column of the excel file, we typed = Rand (), by pressing enter a decimal number appeared. We included the whole multitude of records, and then we sorted through the column we created, from smallest to largest. This created the 3rd test set file.

At this point, since we had already created all the files, we proceeded to examine each set individually (1st training set with 1st test set, 2nd training set with 2nd test set, 3rd training set with 3rd test set), in order to decide, which one we will use, based on the accuracy rate and the decision tree that gave us.

By checking the three different cases we noticed that we had the best results in the third case and then in the first case. At this point, in order to improve the results of both the 3rd and the 1st set, we identified the number of items that were incorrectly categorized as false negatives and then gradually removed them, checking each time the change that resulted in the accuracy rate of the system as well as the decision tree. This was done to further increase the reliability of our model.

We finally achieved, using the 3rd training set and the 3rd test set, with the RANDOMTREE algorithm, an accuracy rate of 83.3%. This was also the ideal set to finally use we adapted to our work.

According to our results we can see that the trained intelligent system based on patient education data included in this study has a high performance. This means that for each new patient it can be reliably predicted whether or not we will have an endoleak.

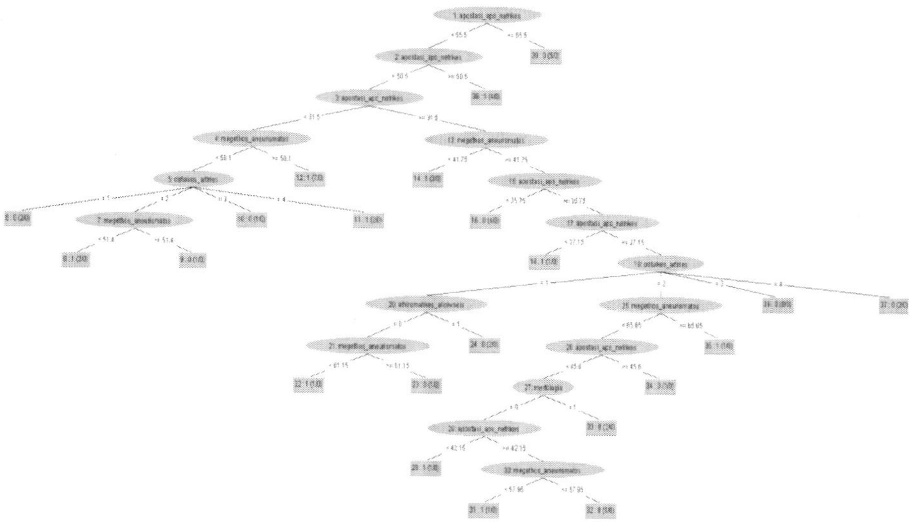

Figure 3. WEKA Decision Tree output.

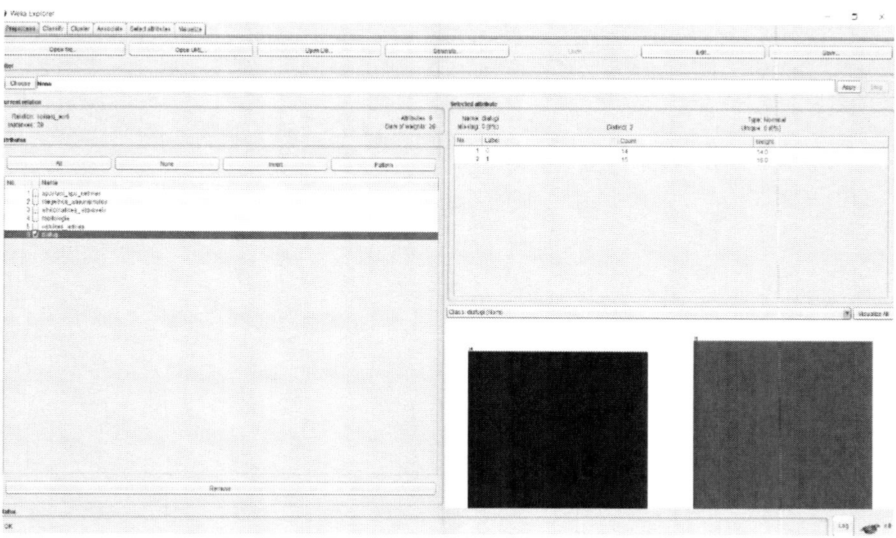

Figure 4. Data presentation.

```
=== Summary ===

Correctly Classified Instances          10               83.3333 %
Incorrectly Classified Instances         2               16.6667 %
Kappa statistic                          0.6667
Mean absolute error                      0.1667
Root mean squared error                  0.4082
Relative absolute error                 33.6957 %
Root relative squared error             82.4982 %
Total Number of Instances               12

=== Detailed Accuracy By Class ===

                 TP Rate  FP Rate  Precision  Recall   F-Measure  MCC      ROC Area  PRC Area  Class
                 1,000    0,250    0,667      1,000    0,800      0,707    0,875     0,667     0
                 0,750    0,000    1,000      0,750    0,857      0,707    0,875     0,917     1
Weighted Avg.    0,833    0,083    0,889      0,833    0,838      0,707    0,875     0,833

=== Confusion Matrix ===

 a b   <-- classified as
 4 0 | a = 0
 2 6 | b = 1
```

Figure 5. Algorithm classificaion results.

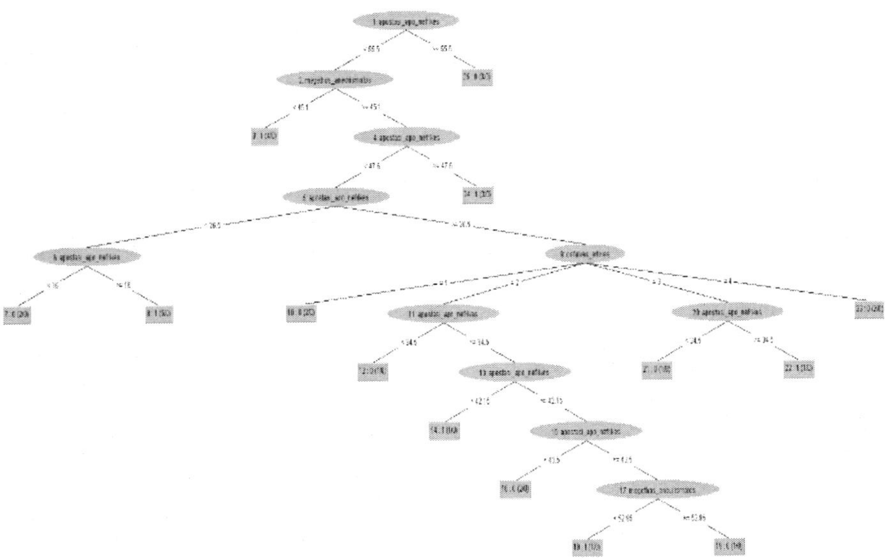

Figure 6. Prognosis classification results.

Table 1. Part of the training data set

```
apostasi_apo_nefrikes,megethos_aneurismatos,
athiromatikes_alloiwseis,morfologia,
osfuikes_artiries,diafugi


56.3,63,1,0,3,0
27,57.7,1,1,2,0
26,63.5,0,0,3,1
15,54.1,1,0,1,0
35.3,50,1,0,1,0
35.5,52.1,1,0,4,0
34,41,0,0,2,1
25.6,58.9,0,0,3,1
33,75.8,0,1,3,0
62,57.6,0,0,3,0
```

Discussion

AI has demonstrated superiority over linear statistical models in previous reports from the medical field [20, 21]. The experience of using A.I. such as its prognostic and diagnostic value in acute pancreatitis and pancreatic cancer has shown that the treatment of such disorders could be significantly improved by these prognostic systems. There are many medical applications for the literature, for example, artificial neural networks in the literature, including predicting cancer survival, predicting outcomes in patients with colorectal diseases, staging and image analysis in non-small cell carcinoma and cancer. It has been widely used in predicting mortality and therapeutic outcomes in elderly patients undergoing hip fractures and neurological diseases such as Alzheimer's disease and other cognitive disorders [28].

Concerning our research and to our knowledge, this is the first study to evaluate the predictive value of CT techniques based on CTA images for preoperative mapping and to provide clinicians with useful information as to whether an aneurysm should be left in the anus abdominal aorta.

In our project, we used five data mining algorithms available in the WEKA software tool. Although the results of all the algorithms were satisfactory, the Random Tree algorithm produced the best results. According to the mathematical approach, it can only be explained by the type and structure of our data. Most patient data could result in faster or even different algorithmic performances between data mining techniques.

Despite the effectiveness of the above models, there are some limitations that need to be improved to be more precise, as it sometimes seems that the model incorrectly classifies some of the data. This can be attributed to the fact that the choice of an acceptable error rate, as well as the choice between false positive or false negative, depending on the creator of the model who sometimes cannot distinguish them.

This study reveals that the most important application of AI is in extremely complex medical situations where prognostic factors and their relationships, which may influence treatment decisions, are not detectable in most common statistical algorithms. Software tools, such as WEKA, usually include A.I. as well as statistical approaches that the user could compare to get the best performance [22, 23, 28].

CONCLUSION AND FUTURE PROSPECTS

The prediction of endoleak into the abdominal aortic aneurysm sac is dependent on imaging studies. Using artificial intelligence tools in clinical practice can prove to be beneficial as it could make it easier for health professionals to make useful and informed medical decisions faster and simpler using mobile applications.

In the future and after collecting a new patient record set the system can update the internal reasoning model, re-calculate its "new performance and give even more accurate results".

REFERENCES

[1] Hirsch AT, Haskal ZJ, Hertzer NR, et al. ACC/AHA 2005 Practice Guidelines for the management of patients with peripheral arterial disease (lower extremity, renal, mesenteric, and abdominal aortic): A collaborative report from the American Association for Vascular Surgery/Society for Vascular Surgery, Society for Cardiovascular Angiography and Interventions, Society for Vascular Medicine and Biology, Society of Interventional Radiology, and the ACC/AHA Task Force on Practice Guidelines (Writing Committee to Develop Guidelines for the Management of Patients With Peripheral Arterial Disease): Endorsed by the American Association of Cardiovascular and Pulmonary Rehabilitation; National Heart, Lung, and Blood Institute; Society for Vascular Nursing; Trans-Atlantic Inter-Society Consensus; and Vascular Disease Foundation. *Circulation.* 2006;113:e463–e654. [PubMed] [Google Scholar].

[2] Ouriel K, Green RM, Donayre C, et al. An evaluation of new methods of expressing aortic aneurysm size: Relationship to rupture. *J. Vasc. Surg*. 1992;15:12-8 [PubMed] [Google Scholar].

[3] Silverberg E, Boring CC, Squires TS. Cancer statistics, 1990. *CA Cancer J. Clin.* 1990;40:9–26.[PubMed] [Google Scholar].

[4] McPhee JT, Hill JS, Eslami MH. The impact of gender on presentation, therapy, and mortality of abdominal aortic aneurysm in the United States, 2001–2004. *J. Vasc. Surg.* 2007;45:891–9. [PubMed] [Google Scholar].

[5] Singh K, Bonaa KH, Jacobsen BK, et al. Prevalence of and risk factors for abdominal aortic aneurysms in a population-based study: The Tromso Study. *Am. J. Epidemiol.* 2001;154:236–44. [PubMed] [Google Scholar].

[6] Kent KC (27 November 2014). "Clinical practice. Abdominal aortic aneurysms". *The New England Journal of Medicine.* 371 (22): 2101–8. doi:10.1056/NEJMcp1401430. PMID 25427112.

[7] Abdominal aortic aneurysm Mayo Clinic https://www.mayoclinic.org/ diseases-conditions/abdominal-aortic-aneurysm/symptoms-causes/syc-203 50688.

[8] Abdominal Aortic Aneurysm Open Repair Stanford Health Care https://stanfordhealthcare.org/medical-conditions/blood-heart-circulation/abdominal-aortic-aneurysm/treatments/abdominal-aortic-aneurysm-open-repair.html.

[9] Open AAA Repair Operation circulation foundation http://www.angionet.gr/en/treatment-therapy/aortic-aneurysm-surgical-repair/.

[10] University of California San Francisco Open Aortic Aneurysm Repair https://surgery.ucsf.edu/conditions--procedures/open-aortic-aneury sm-repair.aspx.

[11] Endovascular Aneurysm Repair University of California San Francisco https://surgery.ucsf.edu/conditions--procedures/endovas cular-aneurysm-repair.aspx.

[12] Endovascular aneurysm repair Greenhalgh RM, Powell JT (2008). "Endovascular repair of abdominal aortic aneurysm". N. Engl. J. Med. 358 (5): 494–501. doi:10.1056/NEJMct0707524. PMID18234 753.

[13] Machine Learning, Wald I, July 2002. http://stat-www.berkeley.edu/users/breiman/wald2002-1.pdf.

[14] Looking Inside the Black Box, Wald II, July 2002. http://stat-www.berkeley.edu/users/breiman/wald2002-2.pdf.

[15] Software for the Masses, Wald III, July 2002. http://stat-www.berkeley. edu/users/breiman/wald2002-3.pdf.

[16] http://www.stat.berkeley.edu/users/breiman/RandomForests/cc_home .htm.

[17] WEKA G. Holmes; A. Donkin; I.H. Witten (1994). "Weka: A machine learning workbench" (PDF). Proc Second Australia and New Zealand Conference on Intelligent Information Systems, Brisbane, Australia. WEKA .Application of artificial neural networks to clinical medicine. *Lancet* 1995q346:1135-1138.

[18] WEKA Machine Learning Group at the University of Waikato: http://www.cs.waikato.ac.nz/ml/index.

[19] Marchevsky AM, Patel S, Wiley KJ, et al. Artificial neural networks and logistic regression as tools for prediction of survival in patients with stages I and II non-small cell lung cancer. *Mod. Patho*l. 1998;11:618-625.

[20] C Koutsojannis, C Lithari, I. Hatzilygeroudis. Managing urinary incontinence through hand-held real-time decision support aid. MEDICON 2010, *IFMBE Proceedings* 29, pp. 913–919, 2010.

[21] Burke HB, Goodman PH, Rosen DB, Henson DE, Weinstein JN, Harrell FE Jr et al. Artificial neural networks improve the accuracy of cancer survival prediction. *Cancer* 1997;79:857-862.

[22] Baxt WG. Application of artificial neural networks to clinical medicine. *Lancet* 1995;346:1135-1138.

[23] Breiman L., Friedman J., Stone C. J., Olshen R. A. (1984). *Classification and Regression Trees*. Boca Raton, FL: CRC press.

[24] Breiman L. (1996). Bagging predictors. *Mach. Learn.* 24, 123–140. 10.1007.

[25] Ceriani L., Verme P. (2012). The origins of the gini index: extracts from variabilità e mutabilità (1912) by corrado gini. *J. Econ. Inequal.* 10, 421–443. 10.1007.

[26] Strobl C., Boulesteix A. L., Augustin T. (2007). Unbiased split selection for classification trees based on the gini index. *Comput. Stat. Data Anal.* 52, 483–501. 10.1016.

[27] Sarica, A., Cerasa, A., & Quattrone, A. (2017). Random Forest Algorithm for the Classification of Neuroimaging Data in Alzheimer's Disease: A Systematic Review. *Frontiers in Aging Neuroscience*, 9, 329.

[28] https://www.nqvascular.com.au/services/aortic-disease/abdominal-thoracic-aortic-aneurysm-s/.

[29] https://www.advancedheartandvein.com/aneurysm-repair.

Biographical Sketches

Chasapi Maria - Constantina

Chasapi Maria - Constantina is currently a Postgraduate student in the Postgraduate Program in Informatics For Life Sciences at the University of Patras. She completed her undergraduate studies at the University of Thessaly, Department of Informatics and Computer Technology. During her thesis, she involved in robotics and in particular the control of a robotic vehicle with Arduino. She has completed her internship at the University of Patras General Hospital "Panayia I Voitheia" in the Department of Networking & Equipment Operation & Management as well as in the Department of Software & Operations Management. She pursued postgraduate studies at the University of Patras, which enabled her to pursue Computer Science in Medical Applications and Artificial Intelligence, where, using Data Mining, knowledge is extracted to assist health professionals in obtaining useful information decisions, faster and simpler. Currently, she is studying endoleak prediction in the abdominal aortic aneurysm, using machine learning algorithms.

Zampakis Peter

Dr Zampakis Peter is Associate Professor of Neuroradiology - Interventional Neuroradiology at University of Patras (UP) Medical School, Patras, Greece. Since 2008, he has officially appointed (by the Ministry of Public Health) as the head person of the Department of Interventional Neuroradiology at the University Hospital of Patras. He teaches Neuroradiology to the Medical students, as well as to post-graduated students in Neuro-Sciences. Regarding his scientific –research work, this is mainly focused on Interventional and Diagnostic Neuroradiology. He has also special interest in the field of Head and Neck radiology. He has published in a number international journals, conferences and books on the fields of his interest.

Constantinos Koutsojannis

Associate Professor, Constantinos Koutsojannis is currently Director of Laboratory of Health Physics & Computational Intelligence, in University of Patras. He is Medical Physicist and expert in Medical Informatics. He is teaching Biophysics, Biostatistics, Research Methodology, Computational Intelligence, Artificial Intelligence and Medical Informatics in several undergraduate and master programs of University of Patras, University of Ioannina and University of Athens. He is involved in a number of Research and Development National and European Projects concerning Artificial Intelligence and serves as a consultant in Artificial Intelligence Working Group as well as full member of Project Committee of European Federation of Medical Physics. His research deals with Biophysics and Medical Applications with Artificial Intelligence on diagnosis, treatment and training using methods of Medical Knowledge representation and extraction from patient data record, medical textbooks and field experts. He has published in a number international journals, conferences and books on the fields of his interest.

In: Medical Knowledge Extraction …
Editor: C. M. Koutsojannis
ISBN: 978-1-53617-925-5

Chapter 6

INTELLIGENT EVALUATION OF MORPHOLOGICAL FACTORS WHICH AFFECT THE MANIFEST OR NOT OF STROKE IN PATIENTS WITH CAROTID DISEASE BY USING DATA MINING ALGORITHMS

***Chasapi Lamprini*[1,*], *Zampakis Petros*[2] *and Constantinos Koutsojannis*[1]**
[1]Laboratory of Health Physics & Computational Intelligence, University Patras, Patras, Greece
[2]Department of Radiology, University of Patras, Patras, Greece

ABSTRACT

The development and evaluation of an intelligent prediction system for the manifest or not of stroke, in patients with carotid disease, based on morphological factors derived from visual data, developed with Machine Learning approaches.

---

* Corresponding Author's Email: lchasapi@upatras.gr.

Data from symptomatic and asymptomatic patients referred to our Hospital University Department of Radiology-Computed Tomography were used in a retrospective chart analysis. Based on simple clinical and CT imaging information and criteria such as CT diagnosis, left or right carotid, rate of stenosis, presence of ulcers, type of atherosclerotic plaque, post-stenotic shrinkage and other vessels, data mining algorithms were constructed.

The final developed computer system based on the Random Tree data mining algorithm predicted the best outcome for all the patients, symptomatic or asymptomatic.

The intelligent approach revealed better performance than the commonly used only imaging criteria in predicting whether or not a stroke occurs, in patients with carotid disease.

Keywords: CT imaging, carotid disease, symptomatic, asymptomatic, machine learning, intelligent prediction system, stroke

Introduction

The Carotid Disease

The carotid arteries are branches of the aorta that carry oxygen-rich blood and nutrients from the heart to the head and the rest of the body. There are two carotid arteries (one on each side of the throat), responsible for the blood supply to the anterior part of the brain. Normally, the inside of the carotid wall is smooth, but over time, an abnormal projection may form, called an atherosclerotic plaque (Figure 1). This plaque is composed of cholesterol, calcium and fibrous tissue and can lead to stenosis or even blockage of the carotid artery. More specifically, carotid disease (or carotid disease) is called stenosis or occlusion of the carotid arteries. The development of the carotid disease can lead to a significant narrowing of the lumen or rupture of the atherosclerotic plaque and release of thrombotic material that can result in blood flow to the smaller arteries of the brain and block them [3, 9]. This results in a decrease or disruption of blood flow and consequently oxygen to the brain, leading to "asphyxiation" and ultimately destruction of brain cells with a potential risk of a stroke. Therefore, ischemic stroke [4] when the brain injury is the permanent, or transient ischemic episode when the disorder of the brain is temporary.

Atherosclerosis is the major risk factor for the development of carotid disease. Arterial hypertension, hyperlipidemia, hypercholesterolemia, diabetes mellitus, smoking, obesity, sedentary life, adulthood, stress, familial predisposition, genetic factors and anatomical variations in Will's cycle, form the predisposing factors for the disease [1]. As a result, we have a hemorrhagic stroke which is mostly related to hypertension and ischemic stroke which is often associated with atherosclerosis [1, 4, 7].

Carotid disease is most commonly found in the division of the common carotid artery and the first centimeters of the internal carotid artery. Less common is the appearance of the common carotid artery.

If the carotid stenosis is not significant, it may present no symptoms in the early stages [7]. The first sign of the disease can be a severe stroke with permanent effects on the brain function, which shows symptomatic stenosis [7, 8, 9, 10]. However, there may be some warning symptoms of stroke, such as transient ischemic attack (PI). The characteristic feature of transient ischemic episodes is that the symptoms resolve completely within 24 hours and the symptoms that can occur are [7, 9, 10]:

- Movement disorders with an opposite or upper limb or facial hemispheres.
- Lack of orientation, headache, confusion.
- Aesthetic disorders with hypersensitivity of the opposite side of the upper or lower limb or face.
- Abnormal disorders that affect the center of speech in the brain, resulting in either confused speech or loss of speech.
- Visual disorders when plaque or thrombus debris enters the artery of the eyes, resulting in sudden temporary blindness called amaurosis fugax and lasts for a few seconds.

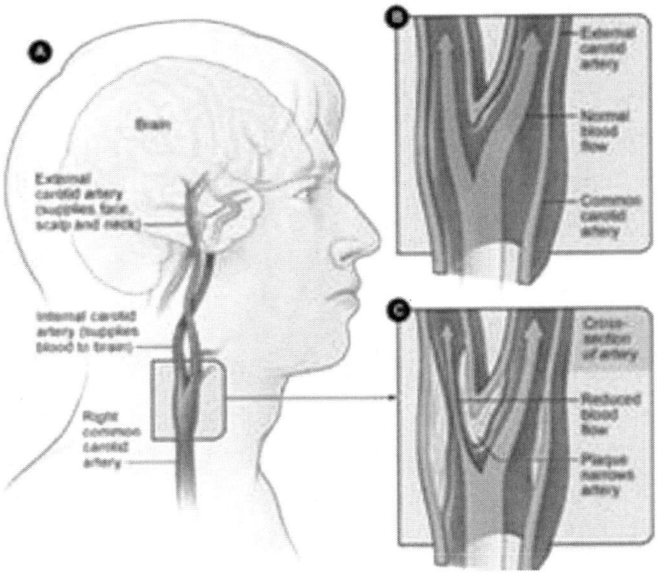

Figure 1. Figure A shows the location of the right carotid artery in the head and neck. Figure B shows the inside of a normal carotid artery that has normal blood flow. Figure C shows the inside of a carotid artery that has plaque buildup and reduced blood flow. Carotid artery disease is serious because it can cause a stroke, also called a "brain attack." A stroke occurs if blood flow to your brain is cut off. If blood flow is cut off, for more than a few minutes, the cells in the brain start to die. This impairs the parts of the body that the brain cells control. A stroke can cause lasting brain damage; long-term disability, such as vision or speech problems or paralysis (an inability to move), or death (modified Figure 1) [25].

There are many ways of imaging the diagnosis of carotid disease. One way is

Carotid Triplex Colour Flow Ultrasound

It is a safe and painless method of imaging and diagnosing the disease that combines ultrasound imaging with the analysis of blood flow velocity at the point of stenosis. It assesses stenosis or obstruction in carotid bifurcation, as it studies the existence and extent of atherosclerotic plaques and whether they can cause significant obstruction. It gives important information on the texture and stability of the plate. Based on the findings from the carotid artery study, patients may need to be appropriately treated or may have to undergo carotid artery surgery [2, 8].

The main imaging test for the diagnosis of the carotid disease is:

Carotid Axial Angiography (CTA)

The CTA is the main objective diagnostic test used in daily practice and is performed with computed tomography and intravenous injection of a contrast medium to produce detailed images of the arteries [2, 8]. It is a convenient method for calculating the degree of carotid stenosis since it is an extremely fast method capable of visualizing the entire vascular tree from the aortic arch to the Willis circle in just 5 seconds and provides better spatial resolution. It is capable of identifying and evaluating the severity of the stenosis since it identifies lesions that have not been adequately evaluated by ultrasound. It depicts vascular calcifications throughout, distinguishes the soft plate and calcifications. Through the development of technology, multisomic tomographs were developed which developed the CTA method. The CTA offers angiographic quality and provides information on the atherosclerotic wall, allowing it to be controlled beyond the lumen and to structures outside the vessels, with the possibility of studying the vessels from many different angles. This method reduced the time of the examination, improved the quality of the radiological image, increased the resolution of the image, resulting in better and more timely diagnosis of the disease. It has been found that CTA has a sensitivity of 99%, a specificity of 95.2%, and a success of 98.3%. Alternatively, the cartridge triplex is used [8, 9, 10].

The purpose of this work is to prove the role of Artificial Intelligence (A.I.) techniques and their ability to predict and prevent serious events and illnesses A.I. In particular, it demonstrates the role of A.I, combined with the traditional MDCT technique, to predict carotid disease in symptomatic and asymptomatic patients, and to prevent stroke. A.I. is approved as a forceful computational method that may better than statistics describe non-deterministic associations between different parameters in the plethora of medical databases. Machine Learning includes several A.I. approaches, mainly consisted of Data Mining tools, aiming Knowledge extraction from data concerning well-defined instances of a situation. In medicine, medical knowledge extraction is presented as a type of decision tree or production rules.

PATIENTS AND METHODS

Patient Population and Data Collection

A group of the population consisted of 60 men and 11 women referred to our University Department of Radiology, a section of Computed Tomography in the period 2014-2018, for carotid vertebrae CT scanning to reveal carotid pathology and guiding preoperative mapping. From CT imaging we examined some parameters (Table1). CT imaging was performed with a CT system Toshiba 1880, a 16-slice multidetector CT system (GE Lightspeed 16x) and 64-slice multidetector CT system Toshiba-Aquilion Prime). Patients were on a supine position with arms parallel to their bodies. The parameters for each phase for GE Lightspeed were as follows: detector configuration 16x1.25mm; tube rotation time 0.6s; pitch 0.938; 120kVp; and automatic tube current modulation. For Toshiba were as follows: detector configuration 80X0.5mm; tube rotation time 0.5s; pitch 0.813; 100kVp; and automatic tube current modulation. The data was stored in PACS. The detailed study involved the analysis of axial patterns.

Results

To analyze a large amount of the available health records and extract medical knowledge information, a data mining approach is implemented.

Data mining techniques were performed using the WEKA 3.7.8 that is an open software source code tool [11, 12]. WEKA was developed at the University of Waikato in New Zealand; the name stands for Waikato Environment for Knowledge Analysis The system is written in Java and distributed under the terms of the GNU General Public License. It runs on almost any platform and has been tested under Linux, Windows, and Macintosh operating systems and even on a personal digital assistant. It provides a uniform interface to many different learning algorithms, along with methods for pre and post-processing and for evaluating the result of learning schemes on any given dataset [13]. Weka provides implementations of learning algorithms that can be easily applied to the dataset. It also includes a variety of tools for transforming datasets, such as the algorithms. The Weka workbench is a collection of state-of-the-art machine learning algorithms and data pre-processing tools [11, 12, 13]. It provides extensive support for the whole process of experimental data mining, including preparing the input data, evaluating learning schemes statistically, and visualizing the input data and the result of learning. As well as a variety of learning algorithms, it includes a wide range of pre-processing tools. This diverse and comprehensive toolkit is accessed through a common interface so that its users can compare different methods and identify those that are most appropriate for the problem at hand. All algorithms take their input in the form of a single relational table in the ARFF format. The easiest way to use Weka is through a graphical user interface called Explorer. This gives access to all of its facilities using menu selection and form filling. The WEKA software uses well established mathematical algorithms with a number of them resulting in decision trees for data classification [14]. Decision trees can be used either for identifying interesting information or building predictive models as in the present application. A decision tree is a classification tree that functions as a guide to predict based on a series of decisions based on the input data. Specifically, a decision tree is a flowchart (Figure 3, 4) that divides up the data on each branch without losing any of the data (the number of the given total health records remains constant throughout the study) for making a series of decisions. Every time each tree is created as follows:

each branch of the graphical representation displays a step where a decision must be made based on the data of an input parameter to proceed to the next branch of the tree. This process is repeated until a leaf provides the predicted output (if the patient is symptomatic or asymptomatic). Building a decision tree and when it has been grown up to size, an immediate step is required to test the accuracy of the model. From the beginning, the available data were randomly divided into two subsets, a training set that was used to build the decision tree and a test set that was used to evaluate the accuracy of the model. The training set at the present work included 66 percent of the data (43 patients) whereas the remaining randomly divided data were placed in the test set included 33 percent of the data (29 patients). This check is also important since machine learning algorithms present the issue of so-called overfitting that is the situation in which the induction algorithm generates a classification tree that perfectly fits the training data but is not generalizing to other instances not present. If we enter the system new data, the chosen algorithm continues to develop hypotheses reducing error while the prediction of future unknown values usually becomes worse due to increasing the final test set error [12]. The available methods to avoid overfitting are the pre-pruning and the post-pruning that involves reduction size by removing branches with less power to classify the training set. Pre-pruning stops growing the tree before it perfectly classifies the training set, while post-pruning allows the expanding of the tree to perfectly classify the input set and after cutting branches. The second approach is more effective since it is not easy to precisely estimate at what size will stop evolving the decision tree. The dual goal of pruning is to reduce tree complexity and improve prediction by reduction of overfitting and removal of sections that are based on output error. To create a balance, for one tree to be as simple as possible with as few "branches" and "leaves of decision" while at the same time we will be as accurate as possible ensuring that the produced model will accurately predict a future unknown set of patient data [12, 14].

Decision trees are supervised learning algorithms. The main concept, behind decision tree learning, is: starting from the training data, we build a predictive model that is mapped to a tree structure. The target is to achieve perfect classification with a minimal number of decisions, although not always possible due to the inconsistencies in training data. A decision tree learning algorithm will return a prediction model (Figure 3). At the start each level splits the data according to different attributes, the non-leaf nodes are represented by attributes/parameters, and the leaf nodes represent the predicted variable or output [14]. The algorithm for learning decision trees follows the steps:

starting with the sum of training data
select an attribute or a value that gives *"best"* split
create child nodes
recurse on each child using child data until *all examples have the same class or the amount of data is too small or the tree is too large.*

The main challenge while building the tree is to decide on which attribute to split the data at a certain step to have the "best" split. "Entropy" is a measure of the uncertainty contained in a piece of information and is calculated before and after each split. In the training patient dataset, must be selected the parameter that lowers the entropy [14]:

$$Entropy = -pP * log2(pP) -pN * log2(pN)$$

pP – the proportion of positive (training) examples
pN – the proportion of negative (training) examples

For users that are not familiar with the tool to build the decision tree using the WEKA Explorer one can go from the "Preprocess" tab to the "Open file" button and load the "training stall.arrf" file. Then to the "Classify" tab, from the "Classifier" section choose "trees" > "RANDOMFOREST" and pressing Start. For the moment, the platform does not allow the visualization of the RANDOMFOREST generated trees. The J48 decision tree is the Weka implementation of the standard C4.5 algorithm which is the successor of ID3. Weka allows the generation of the visual version of the decision tree for the J48 algorithm. So, from the "Classifier" section select "trees" > "RANDOMTREE". Also, the "-C 0.25 -M 1" options are selected for the algorithm with:

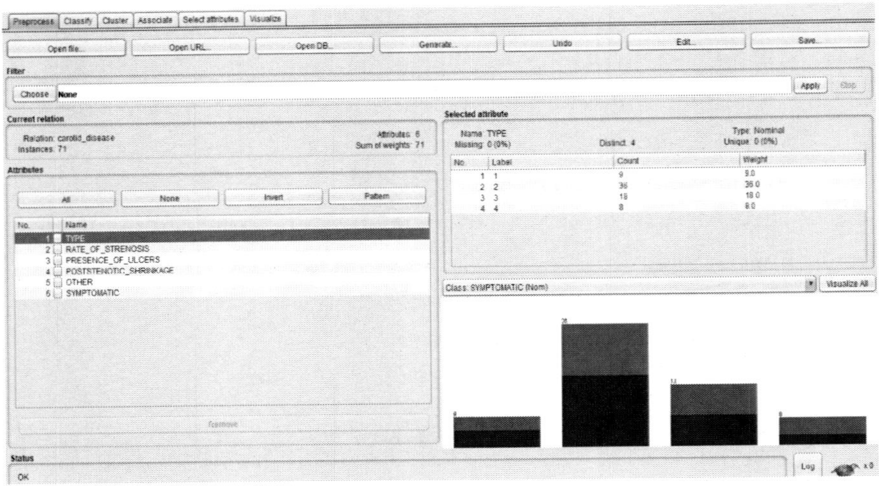

Figure 2. Data presentation.

```
=== Evaluation on test split ===

Time taken to test model on test split: 0.01 seconds

=== Summary ===

Correctly Classified Instances          18               75      %
Incorrectly Classified Instances         6               25      %
Kappa statistic                          0.4419
Mean absolute error                      0.2292
Root mean squared error                  0.4677
Relative absolute error                 45.6007 %
Root relative squared error             93.0486 %
Total Number of Instances               24

=== Detailed Accuracy By Class ===

                 TP Rate  FP Rate  Precision  Recall   F-Measure  MCC      ROC Area  PRC Area  Class
                 0,867    0,444    0,765      0,867    0,813      0,450    0,759     0,788     0
                 0,556    0,133    0,714      0,556    0,625      0,450    0,759     0,605     1
Weighted Avg.    0,750    0,328    0,746      0,750    0,742      0,450    0,759     0,719

=== Confusion Matrix ===

  a  b   <-- classified as
 13  2 |  a = 0
  4  5 |  b = 1
```

Figure 3. Random Tree classification results.

- confidence factor — *The confidence factor used for pruning (smaller values incur more pruning).*
- minNumObj — *The minimum number of instances per leaf.*

Finally pressing "*Start*" the calculation select the result in the left pane, right-click and select the "*Visualize tree*" the final decision tree is created (Figure 4).

The Random Forest Algorithm

The Random Forest (RF) algorithm that has been selected here is a collection or ensemble of Classification and Regression Trees (CART) trained on datasets of the same size as a training set, called bootstraps, created from a random resampling on the training patient data set itself [12, 14]. When the tree is constructed, a set of bootstraps, which do not include any particular record from the original dataset is used as test sets while the error rate of the resulted classification of all the test sets is the estimate of the generalization error. Breiman has proved that, for the bagged classifiers, the error is accurate as using a test set of the same size as the training set. Consequently, using this estimate removes the need for a separate patient data test set. To classify new input data, each CART tree "votes" for one class of output and the "forest" predicts the class that obtains the plurality of all the "votes" [14]. RF has specific rules and is proved robust to overfitting considering more stable in the presence of outliers and very high dimensional parameter spaces than other similar algorithms [18]. The concept of variable importance is an implicit feature selection performed by the RF and assessed by the Gini impurity criterion index [19]. The Gini is a measure of prediction power of all variables in classification, based on the principle of impurity reduction it is non-parametric and therefore does not rely on data belonging to a particular type of distribution [24]. For a split, the Gini index of a node n is:

$$\text{Gini}(n) = 1 - \sum 2\text{j} = 1(\text{pj})2$$

where *pj* is the relative frequency of class j in the node *n*.

For dividing a node in the best way, the improvement in the Gini index should be maximized. In other words, a low Gini means that a specific predictor feature plays a greater role in classifying the patient data into the two classes. Thus, the Gini index can be used to rank the importance of variables for the best classification [12]. We also tested the dataset with alternative knowledge extraction algorithms (as J48, REPTree, Random Tree, RF, LMT) in the form of knowledge decision trees. The following were calculated: sensitivity, specificity, positive prognostic value, and negative prognostic value. Finally, we used the best model according to metrics as sensitivity, specificity, and prognostic value. The best results from our experiments were succeeded with RANDOMTREE algorithms for all the patients.

The Random Tree Algorithm

Random Tree is a supervised Classifier, it is an ensemble learning algorithm that generates many individual learners. It employs a bagging idea to produce a random set of data for constructing a decision tree. In the standard tree, each node is split using the best split among all variables.

In a random forest, each node is split using the best among the subset of predictors randomly chosen at that node. Random trees have been introduced by Leo Breiman and Adele Cutler. The algorithm can deal with both classification and regression problems. Random trees is a collection (ensemble) of tree predictors that is called a *forest*. The classification works as follows: the random trees classifier takes the input feature vector, classifies it with every tree in the forest, and outputs the class label that received the majority of "votes". In the case of a regression, the classifier response is the average of the responses over all the trees in the forest. Random Trees are essentially the combination of two existing algorithms in Machine Learning: single model trees are combined with Random Forest ideas. Model trees are decision trees where every single leaf holds a linear model that is optimized for the local subspace described by this leaf. Random Forests have shown to improve the performance of single decision trees considerably: tree diversity is generated by two ways of randomization. First, the training data is sampled with a replacement for every single tree-like in Bagging. Secondly, when growing a tree, instead of always computing the best possible split for each node only a random subset of all attributes is considered at every node, and the best split for that subset is computed. Such trees have been for classification Random model trees for the first time combine model trees and random forests. Random trees employ this product for split selection and thus induce reasonably balanced trees where one global setting for the ridge value works across all leaves, thus simplifying the optimization procedure. [15, 16, 17].

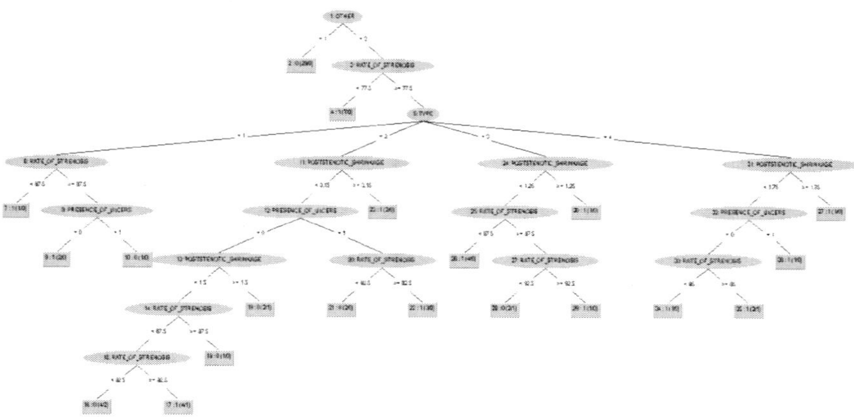

Figure 4. Classification/decision tree.

Table 1. Database's parameters

Input parameters {values}:

@relation carotid_disease

@attribute TYPE {1,2,3,4} based on CT image

@attribute RATE_OF_STRENOSIS real based on CT image

@attribute PRESENCE_OF_ULCERS {0,1} based on CT image

@attribute POSTSTENOTIC_SHRINKAGE real based on CT image

@attribute OTHER {1,2} based on CT image

@attribute SYMPTOMATIC {0,1}

Output parameters {values}:

RESULTS with categorical values {symptomatic or asymptomatic}

Discussion

AI has proven superiority over linear statistical models in previous reports from the medical field [20, 21]. Experience from the use of A.I. such as its prognostic and diagnostic value in acute pancreatitis and pancreatic cancer showed that the management of these kinds of disorders could be greatly improved from these predictive systems [22, 23]. To elaborate there are many medical applications of for example of Artificial Neural Networks in bibliography including cancer survival prediction, outcome prediction in patients suffering from colorectal, staging and image analysis in non-small lung cell carcinoma and breast cancer [22, 23].

A.I. has been also widely used in the prediction of mortality and treatment outcomes in an elderly population undergoing surgery for hip fractures [23] and age-associated neurological diseases such as Alzheimer's disease [23] and other cognitive impairments.

Concerning our research, and according to our knowledge this is the first study that evaluates the prognostic value of AI techniques based on CT images for preoperative mapping and offering clinicians useful information for the outcome or a decision support system that tells us according to the rate of narrowing of the carotid artery, if the symptomatic or asymptomatic patient is about to have a stroke, to be avoided.

In our work, we used five data mining algorithms available at the WEKA software tool. Nevertheless, the results of all algorithms were satisfactory, but the Random Tree algorithm yielded the best results. According to their mathematical approach, it can be explained only from the type and structure of our data [11]. More patient data could result in faster or even different algorithm performances among data mining techniques.

Despite the effectiveness of the above models, there are some limitations [12] that need to be improved to be more accurate as it seems that sometimes the model incorrectly classifies some of the data. This may be attributed to the fact that the choice of an acceptable percentage of errors as the choice between false positive or false negative option depends on the model creator that sometimes cannot distinguish them.

This study reveals that the most important application of AI is in extremely complex medical situations where the prognostic factors and their relationships, are not detectable in most common statistic algorithms [23]. Software tools as WEKA usually include A.I. as well as statistical approaches that the user could compare to have the best output [22, 14].

CONCLUSION

Adjusting an application of A.I. in clinical practice can be demonstrated beneficial as it could facilitate health professionals in taking critical and evidence-based medical decisions provided through fast and simply used as mobile applications.

In the future and after the collection of a new group of patient records the system can update the internal reasoning model, recalculate its' new performance and give even more accurate results [14].

REFERENCES

[1] Doonan, RJ; Abdullah, A; Steinmetz-Wood, S; Mekhaiel, S; Steinmetz, OK; Obrand, DI; Corriveau, MM; Mackenzie, KS; Gill, HL. Carotid Endarterectomy Outcomes in the Elderly: A Canadian Institutional Experience. *Ann Vasc Surg.*, 2019, Feb 22, [PubMed].

[2] Morales, MM; Anacleto, A; Filho, CM; Ledesma, S; Aldrovani, M; Wolosker, N. Peak Systolic Velocity for Calcified Plaques Fails to Estimate Carotid Stenosis Degree. *Ann Vasc Surg.*, 2019 Feb 22, [PubMed].

[3] Savardekar, AR; Narayan, V; Patra, DP; Spetzler, RF; Sun, H. Timing of Carotid Endarterectomy for Symptomatic Carotid Stenosis: A Snapshot of Current Trends and Systematic Review of Literature on Changing Paradigm towards Early Surgery. *Neurosurgery.*, 2019, Feb 25, [PubMed].

[4] Coelho, AP; Lobo, M; Nogueira, C; Gouveia, R; Campos, J; Augusto, R; Coelho, N; Semião, AC; Canedo, A. Overview of evidence on risk factors and early management of acute carotid stent thrombosis during the last two decades. *J. Vasc. Surg.*, 2019 Mar, 69(3), 952-964. [PubMed].

[5] Texakalidis, P; Chaitidis, N; Giannopoulos, S; Giannopoulos, S; Machinis, T; Jabbour, P; Rivet, D; Reavey-Cantwell, J; Rangel-Castilla, L. Carotid Revascularization in Older Adults: A Systematic Review and Meta-Analysis. *World Neurosurg.*, 2019 Feb, 22, [PubMed].

[6] Tokugawa, J; Kudo, K; Mitsuhashi, T; Yanagisawa, N; Nojiri, S; Hishii, M. Surgical Results of Carotid Endarterectomy for Twisted Carotid Bifurcation. *World Neurosurg.*, 2019, Feb 19, [PubMed].

[7] Carotid artery disease Mayo Clinic https://www.mayoclinic.org/diseases-conditions/carotid-artery-disease/symptoms-causes/syc-20360519.

[8] https://www.mayoclinic.org/diseases-conditions/carotid-artery-disease/diagnosis-treatment/drc-20360527.

[9] Carotid Artery Disease: Causes, Symptoms, Tests and Treatment WebMd https://www.webmd.com/heart-disease/carotid-artery-disease-causes-symptoms-tests-and-treatment#1.

[10] Carotid Artery Stenosis https://medlineplus.gov/ency/article/007427.htm.

[11] NHBLI Carotid Artery Disease https://www.nhlbi.nih.gov/health-topics/carotid-artery-disease.

[12] WEKA. Application of artificial neural networks to clinical medicine. *Lancet*, 1995, q. 346, 1135-1138.

[13] WEKA Machine Learning Group at the University of Waikato: http://www.cs.waikato.ac.nz/ml/index.

[14] *International Journal of Emerging Technology and Advanced Engineering* Website: www.ijetae.com (ISSN 2250-2459, ISO 9001, 2008 Certified Journal, Volume 5, Issue 1, January 2015). Comparative Analysis of WEKA Data Mining Algorithm RandomForest, RandomTree, and LADTree for Classification of

Indigenous News Data. Sushilkumar Rameshpant Kalmegh Associate Professor, Department of Computer Science, SGBAU, Amravati (M.S.), India.

[15] Sarica, A; Cerasa, A; Quattrone, A. Random Forest Algorithm for the Classification of Neuroimaging Data in Alzheimer's Disease: A Systematic Review. *Frontiers in Aging Neuroscience*, (2017), 9, 329.

[16] Syed Shajahaan, S; Shanthi, S; ManoChitra, V. "Application of Data Mining Techniques to Model Breast Cancer Data", *International Journal of Emerging Technology and Advanced Engineering*, Volume 3, Issue 11, November 2013, pp- 362-369.

[17] http://www.uetpeshawar.edu.pk/TRP-G/Dr.Nasir-Ahmad-TRP/Journals/2012/Random%20Forests%20and%20Decision%20Trees.pdf.

[18] Bernhard Pfahringer, "Random model trees: an e_ective and scalable regression method" University of Waikato, New Zealand, http://www.cs.waikato.ac.nz/~bernhard.

[19] Breiman, L. Bagging predictors. *Mach. Learn.*, (1996), 24, 123–140. 10.1007.

[20] Ceriani, L; Verme, P. The origins of the gini index: extracts from variabilità e mutabilità (1912) by corrado gini. *J. Econ. Inequal.*, (2012), 10, 421–443, 10.1007.

[21] Marchevsky, AM; Patel, S; Wiley, KJ; et al. Artificial neural networks and logistic regression as tools for prediction of survival in patients with stages I and II non-small cell lung cancer. *Mod Pathol*, 1998, 11, 618-625.

[22] Koutsojannis, C; Lithari, C; Hatzilygeroudis, I. Managing urinary incontinence through hand-held real-time decision support aid. MEDICON 2010, *IFMBE Proceedings*, 29, pp. 913–919, 2010.

[23] Burke, HB; Goodman, PH; Rosen, DB; Henson, DE; Weinstein, JN; Harrell, FE; Jr. et al. Artificial neural networks improve the accuracy of cancer survival prediction. *Cancer*, 1997, 79, 857-862.

[24] Baxt, WG. Application of artificial neural networks to clinical medicine. *Lancet*, 1995, 346, 1135-1138.

[25] Strobl, C; Boulesteix, AL; Augustin, T. Unbiased split selection for classification trees based on the gini index. *Comput. Stat. Data Anal.*, (2007), 52, 483–501, 10.1016.
[26] Carotid Arteries Image https://www.nhlbi.nih.gov/health-topics/carotid-artery-disease.

Biographical Sketches

Chasapi Lamprini

Chasapi Lamprini, is currently a Postgraduate student in the Postgraduate Program in Informatics for Life Sciences at the University of Patras. She was born and raised in Athens. She has successfully completed her undergraduate studies at the University of Thessaly, Department of Computer Engineering and Computer Technology, completing her bachelor's thesis on Arduino and in particular robotic vehicle control using Arduino. She has been working as a Computer Engineer in the Computer Engineering Department of Hellenic Aerospace Industry, in Schimatari, Boeotia, as part of her internship. She is currently, a postgraduate student of Medical School in the program of Informatics for Life Sciences, at the University of Patras while carrying out her diplomatic work, she deals with Data Mining Algorithms where useful tools for the detection or not of stroke in patients with carotid disease are extracted through Artificial Intelligence tools.

Zampakis Petros

Dr Zampakis Petros is Associate Professor of Neuroradiology - Interventional Neuroradiology at University of Patras (UP) Medical School, Patras, Greece. Since 2008, he has officially appointed (by the Ministry of Public Health) as the head person of the Department of Interventional Neuroradiology at the University Hospital of Patras. He teaches Neuroradiology to the Medical students, as well as to post-graduated students in Neuro-Sciences. Regarding his scientific –research work, this is mainly focused on Interventional and Diagnostic Neuroradiology. He has also special interest in the field of Head and Neck radiology. He has published in a number international journals, conferences and books on the fields of his interest.

Constantinos Koutsojannis

Associate Professor, Constantinos Koutsojannis is currently Director of Laboratory of Health Physics & Computational Intelligence, in University of Patras. He is Medical Physicist and expert in Medical Informatics. He is teaching Biophysics, Biostatistics, Research Methodology, Computational Intelligence, Artificial Intelligence and Medical Informatics in several undergraduate and master programs of University of Patras, University of Ioannina and University of Athens. He is involved in a number of Research and Development National and European Projects concerning Artificial Intelligence and serves as a consultant in Artificial Intelligence Working Group as well as full member of Project Committee of European Federation of Medical Physics. His research deals with Biophysics and Medical Applications with Artificial Intelligence on diagnosis, treatment and training using methods of Medical Knowledge representation and extraction from patient data record, medical textbooks and field experts. He has published in a number international journals, conferences and books on the fields of his interest.

In: Medical Knowledge Extraction …
Editor: C. M. Koutsojannis
ISBN: 978-1-53617-925-5

Chapter 7

General Knowledge Modified from Expert's Clinical Experience for Precise Depression Diagnosis in a Mobile Intelligent System

Andreas Andrikopoulos[1,*], PhD,
Constantinos Koutsojannis[1], PhD
and Ioannis Hatzilygeroudis[2], PhD
[1]Laboratory of Health Physics & Computational Intelligence, University of Patras, Patras, Greece
[2]Computer Engineering & Informatics Department University of Patras, Patras, Greece

Abstract

Depression is the most common mental illness with which it confronts both the psychiatrists and specific health professionals. This disease adds a large impact on the psychological and economic condition

---

* Corresponding Author's Email: anandrikop@gmail.com.

of patients, their families, and the community. The detection of stages of depression is crucial not only for experts to choose efficient treatment and support of patients but also for the people close to the patient. Several established questionnaires are already used to support experts' experience which is shifting to its' interpersonal dialog-based ability as the professional time passes. In this paper, we present an intelligent system for depression diagnosis that aims to assist the interfering health professionals in decision making. This computer diagnosis process is based on an expert system module that was developed using the expert's experience, fused with the analysis of the questionnaire's results representing the general knowledge taking into account successful examples from clinical practice.

The system takes as input parameters sleep, behavior, mood as well as thoughts and feelings, motility and physical condition as results of established tools. Afterward, the system outputs the possible diagnosis if depression exists or not as well as it categorizes it in seven internationally established types. An evaluation study was conducted to modify the "by the book" internal reasoning as well as to assess the system's performance and the results are very encouraging providing high precision. This system as a mobile application can alternatively be used for decision support of doctor residents or early detection of a person's abnormal behavior from members of the close community as social volunteers and even relatives.

Keywords: depression diagnosis, expert system, patient behavior analysis

INTRODUCTION

In mental health, emotional disorders are of particular interest. Depression is an emotional state of intense and persistent sadness [1]. It may range from mild sadness to extreme despair, one of the most common mental health problems [1, 2]. The term depression in psychiatry suggests a disorder that has a combination of symptoms. One of the most common symptoms of depression is the bad mood but it is not the only one, and there are types of the disorder that is not detected [3]. The importance of depression is not only to a large extent of the people who suffer, but it must also be taken into account the great risk of self-destruction resulting from it, the impact on family and work and the economic impact (i.e., early retirement, productivity impact) [4]. Their diagnosis, however, is extremely difficult. On the one hand due to polymorphic presentations, on the other hand, due to confusion with severe symptomatic situations, such as behavioral disorders, addictive disorders, and schizophrenic disorders. Depression is believed to be autonomous and only slightly affected by events and existential conditions (although early illnesses often follow splitting or loss) [3, 5]. Therefore, the diagnosis of depression faces particular difficulties. The diagnosis of an episode of depression in the first one of some complete diagnosis steps that comprise the definition of the elements, which together with the melancholic and informal features characterize the episode [4, 6, 7]. Additionally, specific types of mood disorders should be considered. Some of these subtype categories meet the internationally accepted criteria of the DSM-IV-TR questionnaire (REFERENCE) for mood disorders with or without specific symptoms or determinants of the course of the disease, and some are often syndromes that may not meet the standard diagnostic criteria but have an undeniable clinical significance [3, 8, 9, 10].

Knowledge Discovery (KD) is the process of extracting information from a large volume of data. A multi-disciplinary field of science and technology, includes statistics, database systems, computer programming, machine learning, and Artificial Intelligence (AI). Knowledge is at the heart of healthcare processes and comes in various forms: definitions of medical terms, relationships between symptoms and diseases, guidelines for treating patients, models for making rational decisions, etc. These essential issues involve the nature of medical knowledge, medical guidelines, and assessment of AI employment in healthcare decision making. Machine Learning (ML) includes many Artificial Intelligence approaches mainly consisting of Data Mining (DM) tools aiming KD from data concerning well-defined instances of a situation. In medicine medical knowledge extraction as a type of decision tree or production rules [11, 12].

Consequently in this paper, we introduce an approach of developing a medical intelligent system based on knowledge extraction from the patient record database that reflects experts' experience, working in a closed psychiatric department of the Greek public mental disorder network in Western Greece, closely combined with the "*by the book*" approach based on internationally established questionnaires [10, 11]. The result is an intelligent system for the diagnosis of depression with the required certification of an established diagnostics tool that has been used in paper form, by experts and includes the general knowledge as is used by them in the real clinical environment. The operation of the expert computer tool mentioned above can be used not competing but complementary to the success of greater reliability but also for the rapid and reliable screening and diagnosis of the diseases of patients with a possible neuropsychiatric disorder. An extensive and evaluated overview of the present system would be applied to the clinical practice with the main focus on the education of all categories of health care professions interacting with the specific field.

The rest of the paper is organized as follows: Section II presents background topics on recognition of depression and describes related works. Section III illustrates the modeling of the diagnosis process and the intelligent system formulated. Section IV presents the experimental study conducted and the results gathered. Finally, Section V concludes the paper and provides directions for future work.

RELATED WORK

The presentation of medical information is not the only demand. This information nowadays must have a form that allows an effective course of reasoning and conclusions to be drawn for the individual who seeks it [23]. The term expert system (ES) in the field of AI describes computer programs whose main characteristic is the presence of intelligent behavior in specific fields based on well-described reasoning.

Recommendation and advice are the main two characteristics that will corporate with experts in the field of artificial intelligence to lead a non-expert user to have a better aspect in different decision – making [12]. The examination of the components concludes an accurate contribution to the creation of an ES. Interference rules that come of applied knowledge of physician results in a positive leveling of documented clinical diagnosis [13]. In AI, an experienced system is a computing system that mimics the ability of an expert in decision making [14]. ESs were designed to solve complex problems based on the available knowledge in a field, as an expert does, and not by executing a precise resolving procedure that a developer has specified, as in the case of conventional computer programming [15, 16]. An ES benefit is the simplicity and familiar representation of knowledge. This gave a prominent role in various areas of medicine [17]. Several successful systems are already in use in medicine [22, 23. 24]. The ITSB authoring tool is an intelligent teaching system for students learning about diabetes. The intelligent system was developed for students wishing to study medicine or to increase their knowledge [26]. Another work that shows the effectiveness of expert systems, deals with male infertility diseases. Doctors have tested it in patients who suffered from this malady. The efficiency of this system procedure satisfied the physicians with a good rate of results [27].

Over the last years, many researchers have been trying to recognize depression with the help of AI through image or natural language analysis with slight success. However, since the advent of machine learning processes, the results seem to have improved significantly [30]. According to this work, by comparing the brain scans of those affected and those not affected by depression, it was possible to make the right diagnosis with a 74% probability. Machine Learning is now being enlisted in other research to investigate vocal patterns that could signal that someone has post-traumatic stress disorder, for example [31]. Participating in this campaign to involve AI in this field that is mainly based on dialog sessions between the experts and the patients from early diagnosis to treatment and follow up. Today even researchers in electronic social networks are currently experimenting with AI technology, which aims to detect posts that could suggest the user may be suicidal or even abnormal [32]. It is also anticipated that AI technology will in the future be able to help doctors choose the right treatment method for their patients [32]. At Weill Cornell Medical College in New York, machine-learning algorithms have been used to distinguish four different types of depression based on brain scans of depressed patients [32]. In our approach, some machine-learning algorithms were used to deal with patient questionnaire answers combined with the final diagnosis certified by experts to choose the one with the best performance. We hope that in the future this will help doctors make more effective choices in terms of the right therapy and AI can even help provide therapy: further, than Tess, where it was developed a psychologically trained AI chatbot that patients with depression can talk to anytime [33].

DIAGNOSIS PROCESS MODELLING

The term depression in psychiatry suggests a disorder that has a combination of symptoms. One of the characteristics of depression is the bad mood for it and it was named, but it is not the only one, and sometimes it may be absent [4, 20]. The main symptoms of a depressed patient are as follows in Table 1. There is no need to have all the symptoms to be considered depressed. Experts believe that 5 or more symptoms of which at least one of the first is enough to get diagnosed. Also, it should be stressed that depressive emotion is intense, is permanent and not affected by the situations the patient is living with. Also, in depression, feeling may be worse in the morning than in the evening, while normal people who just feel distressed are usually better when they get up in the morning [18, 19].

The three main forms of depression experienced by a depressed patient are as follows: Depression in the context of a unilateral affective disorder (Major Depression) or bipolar affective disorder. Mild or Minor Depression (mild symptoms). Dizziness: when mild or minor depression is delayed for more than 2 years, it changes into a dysthymic disorder. Other types of depression occur in a patient according to some social criteria and have the following forms: anxiety depression, depression with psychotic type movement retardation, reactive depression, neurotic depression, seasonal depression, geriatric depression, etc. Differential diagnosis should be made of grief, mourning, anxiety disorders, schizophrenia, upsets, depression associated with alcoholism [4, 20, 21]. To create an intelligent system for the diagnosis of depression, it is necessary to validate a certified diagnostics tool - a scale that has hitherto been used in paper form by experts and includes the general knowledge as presented in the previous section.

Table 1. Symptoms of depression

A great reduction in interest or pleasure in almost all activities
Depressed mood for most of the day
Ideas of guilt, self-confidence, and worthlessness
Concern and pessimism for the future
Suicide ideas
General bodily symptoms such as headaches, general pain in the body, etc.
Inability to concentrate, think, remember or make decisions
Loss of physical vitality
Loss of interest in erotic action
Disorders of digestive appetite
Difficulties in sleeping

More specifically, it is known that the diagnosis of an episode of mania and depression is the first step for a complete diagnosis. The next steps are to define the elements, which together with the melancholic and informal features characterize the episode. Specific types of mood disorders should then be considered. Some of these subtype categories meet the internationally accepted criteria of the DSM-IV-TR questionnaire for mood disorders with or without specific symptoms or determinants of the course of the disease, and some are often syndromes that may not meet the standard diagnostic criteria but have undoubted clinical significance. For an episode of major depression, a person has to experience at least five of the nine symptoms for over two weeks or more, almost every day during this time, and this is a change from the previous level of activity. One of the symptoms should be either depressed mood or loss of interest (Table 2).

Table 2. General symptoms of depression

The depressed mood on the longest day, almost every day, revealed by either subjective reference (i.e., feeling or void) or by third-party observations (i.e., he/she seems tearful).
Significant weight loss without the restriction of food or weight gain (i.e., change in body weight over 5% in one month) or decrease or increase in appetite almost every day.
Insomnia or drowsiness almost every day
Psychomotor stimulation or slowing almost every day (can be perceived by third parties and is not only a subjective feeling of nervousness or sluggishness)
Fatigue or lack of energy almost every day
A feeling of futility or exaggeration or unwarranted guilt (which may be par aesthetic) almost every day (not only a subjective approach or a sense of guilt for the disease).
The decrease in thinking or concentration or indecision almost every day (either subjective or third-party observation).
Repeated thoughts of death (not just fear of death), recurrent suicidal ideation without a specific plan or attempted suicide, or a specific suicide plan.

Note: Symptoms that are clearly due to pathological conditions or mood-related hallucinations or hallucinations are not included.

We have developed the model of Figure 1 for the diagnosis process of depression that is the most common way that an expert on the field moves from symptoms to a possible diagnosis.

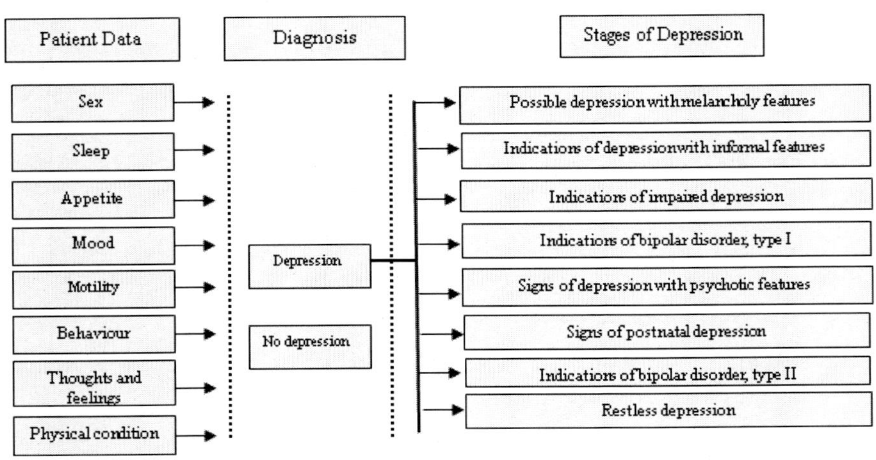

Figure 1. Model of initial and final diagnosis processing.

SYSTEM ARCHITECTURE

To extract knowledge from data, there are used some platforms that provide effective approaches worldwide. WEKA (Waikato Environment for Knowledge Analysis) is one of the most popular knowledge mining software packages from data sets, based on engineering learning algorithms and is written in JAVA programming language [29]. With the help of WEKA tools, we could pre-process the data, sort it and group it, extract correlation rules, create representations (visualized learning outcomes, decision trees), and statistically evaluate the patterns that produced and are presented below in Figure 2, the vertical bold lines indicate inference nodes. According to that, initially, a psychiatrist - psychologist requires the following information: (a) sex, (b) sleep, (c) appetite, (d) mood, (e) motility, (f) behavior, (g) thoughts and feelings and (h) physical condition, which can be characterized as obligatory. At this stage, based on them, an initial diagnosis is made, concerning the nature of the cause of the problem. There are two possible initial diagnoses: the cause of the problem is (a) depression and (b) no depression.

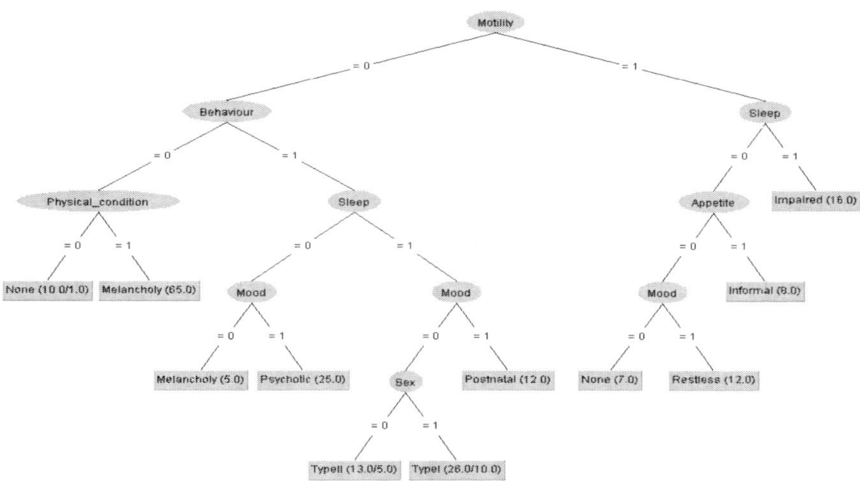

Figure 2. Part of the final diagnosis process for depression as a decision tree.

To confirm and/or further specialize the initial diagnosis, the expert requires further information related to diagnostic laboratory tests that could be characterized as advanced. Once the expert gets results of them, may give a final diagnosis, which can be, (a) possible depression with melancholy features (Melancholy), (b) no depression (None), (c) indications of bipolar disorder - type II (TypeII), (d) signs of postnatal depression (Postnatal), (e) signs of depression with psychotic features (Psychotic), (f) indications of bipolar disorder - type I (Type I), (g) indications of impaired depression (Impaired) (h) indications of depression with informal features (Informal) and finally (i) restless depression (Restless). Based on our expert psychiatrists - psychologists, we specified a set of parameters for each of the entities in the process model that represent patient data (Figure 3) that play a role in diagnosis.

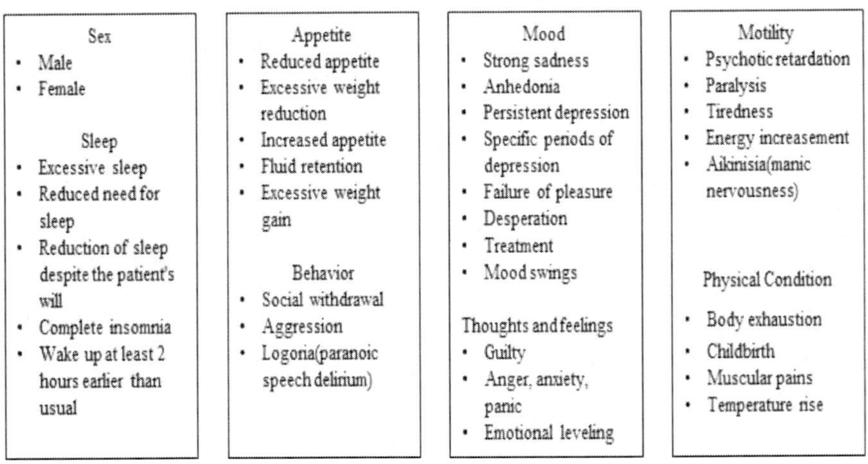

Figure 3. Parameters for each of the entities in the process model that represent patient data.

The patient has to answer a questionnaire after carefully reading the complete instructions and its implementation restrictions. The questionnaire is addressed to adults (excluding children, adolescents, and elders), does not refer to cases of use of addictive substances, mourning, grief accompanied by severe diseases, such as cancer. It also does not concern cases of pathological conditions that may be associated with some of the symptoms of depression. It is important to stress that the questionnaire does not contain validity scales (as in MMPI) [25].

- Input parameters:

Age, Sex, and outputs of specific questionnaires for Sleep, Mood, Appetite, Motility, Behavior, Thoughts and Feelings and Physical Condition (Figure 1) with values "normal" or "abnormal."

- Intermediate parameters:

Possible diagnosis with values: "depression" and "no depression."

- Output parameters:

Final diagnosis with values: (a) possible depression with melancholy features, (b) no depression, (c) indications of bipolar disorder - type II, (d) signs of postnatal depression, (e) signs of depression with psychotic features, (f) indications of bipolar disorder - type I, (g) indications of impaired depression, (h) indications of depression with informal features and (i) restless depression. There are instances where the user attempts to present a different picture than the actual or is not aware of his real image. It is therefore assumed that the user will understand and answer honestly all the questions. It is also stressed that this is a test that is not a formal medical opinion. The medical records of 400 patients who have been visited the emergency department with possible depression symptoms or suspected behavioral disorders were used.

The database included patients from the beginning of 2015 to June 2018. These patients have relapsed in their psychiatric medical record and the rest of them were examined in the context of an integrated medical examination (including psychiatric examination) conducted at the emergency department. In more detail, some patients had a psychiatric medical record and some others were examined by the psychiatrist due to referral from another medical specialty. Of these 400 patients, 196 were men and 204 women. The average age of 40 years with the age being at a minimum of 19 years and a maximum of 75. The data was anonymous and all patients agreed to participate in the recording. 144 of these 400 patients who responded to the questionnaire as presented above were diagnosed with possible depression with melancholy features, 16 were diagnosed with indications of depression with informal features, 32 had evidence of disturbed depression, 36 had evidence of bipolar Type II disorder, 42 had evidence of bipolar disorder Type I disorder, 50 had evidence of depression with psychotic features, 24 had evidence of postnatal depression and 24 had restless depression [28]. The remaining 32 who did not show signs of depression did not show any history of depression during their lifetime. According to the model, we distinguish between input, intermediate and final parameters.

Evaluation Results

There are instances where the user attempts to present a different picture than the actual or is not aware of his real image. It is therefore assumed that the user will understand and answer honestly all the questions. It is also stressed that this is a test that is not a formal medical opinion. There were used the medical records of 400 patients who have been visited the emergency department with possible depression symptoms or suspected behavioral disorders. The database included patients from the beginning of 2015 to June 2018. These patients have relapsed in their psychiatric medical record and the rest of them were examined in the context of an integrated medical examination (including psychiatric examination) conducted at the emergency department. In more detail, some patients had a psychiatric medical record and some others were examined by the psychiatrist due to referral from another medical specialty. Of these 400 patients, 196 were men and 204 women. The average age of 40 years with the age being at a minimum of 19 years and a maximum of 75. The data was anonymous and all patients agreed to participate in the recording. 144 of these 400 patients who responded to the questionnaire as presented above were diagnosed with possible depression with melancholy features, 16 were diagnosed with indications of depression with informal features, 32 had evidence of disturbed depression, 36 had evidence of bipolar Type II disorder, 42 had evidence of bipolar disorder Type I disorder, 50 had evidence of depression with psychotic features, 24 had evidence of postnatal depression and 24 had restless depression [28]. The remaining 32 who did not show signs of depression did not show any history of depression during their lifetime. According to the model, we distinguish between input, intermediate and final parameters. The evaluation study was conducted to assess the ES and provide an insight into its performance. The study concerns the evaluation of the performance of the system in determining accurately the final depression diagnosis. In the context of the study, a dataset of patient records that had their diagnosis determined by experts was used and the performance of the system was specified. More specifically, the dataset consisted of 400 records. Given that we have a multiple class output, we use the following metrics: average accuracy, precision, and F-measure. In general, for a given class, the precision metric is the fraction of the instances that were classified to that class and belong to the class, while recall is the fraction of instances that belong to class A that were correctly classified to that class. The F-measure metric combines the recall and precision values and is calculated as follows:

$$f\_measure = \frac{2 \times prec \times rec}{prec + rec}$$

Finally, the weighted average of these metrics for all classes can be calculated, taking into account the number of occurrences of each class in the dataset. These metrics are widely used in classification performance evaluations and using them allows direct comparison with various classification models. In Table 3, we present the results collected from the evaluation of the ES. The well-known algorithm J48, succeeded the best results among other competitive approaches as LMT, RandomForest, RandomTree, etc.

These results revealed an excellent precision performance of the system even for the most difficult outputs as the correctly classified instances were at the level of 92% for each test set of records (Table 3). The lowest value of precision resulted in the "indications of bipolar disorder - type II" type of depression diagnosis (89%).

Table 3. Evaluation results of the ES

Class	Precision	Recall	F-Measure
Possible depression with melancholy features	1	1	1
No depression	1	1	1
Indications of bipolar disorder - type II	0.89	0.96	0.92
Signs of postnatal depression	0.94	0.84	0.89
Signs of depression with psychotic features	1	1	1
Indications of bipolar disorder - type I	0.95	0.95	0.95
Indications of impaired depression	1	1	1
Indications of depression with informal features	1	1	1
Restless depression	1	1	1
Total Correctly Classified patient records		91,9%	

Graphical Abstract [GA]: General description of the present approach for General Knowledge modification from Expert's Clinical Experience in order to succeed precise Depression Diagnosis in a mobile intelligent system.

After the final construction of the decision tree, the final model was build up as a computer application with ACRES v3.0.1 platform that is an ES developing tool. This tool constructs ESs form data and has been developed from AI Group of Computer Engineering Department of the University of Patras [33]. At the end of this procedure, the user can interact with a form that asking for the input parameters of a new patient and giving as an output, using internally the ES, the possible depression type, combined with the appropriate possibility as a percentage (Figure 4).

The final tool can be easily downloaded on a mobile system for fast and on-site use by the health professional. At present, it is used online from mobile phones or PCs (Figure 5). In the future and after the collection of a new group of patient records the system can update the internal reasoning model, recalculate its' new performance and give even more accurate results [34]. The internal model could change both with future changes in general knowledge that will be absorbed in newly established questionnaires, or experts' final approach according to their experience [34].

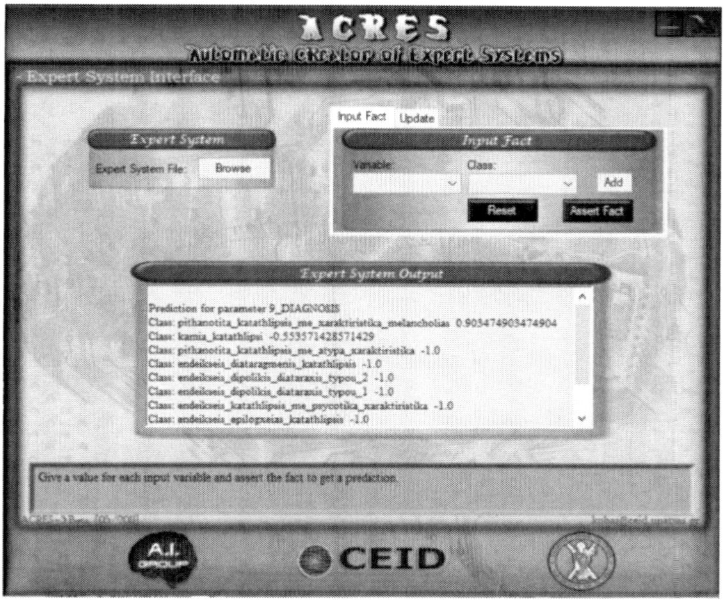

Figure 4. The ACRES v3.0.1 platform for intelligent system creation.

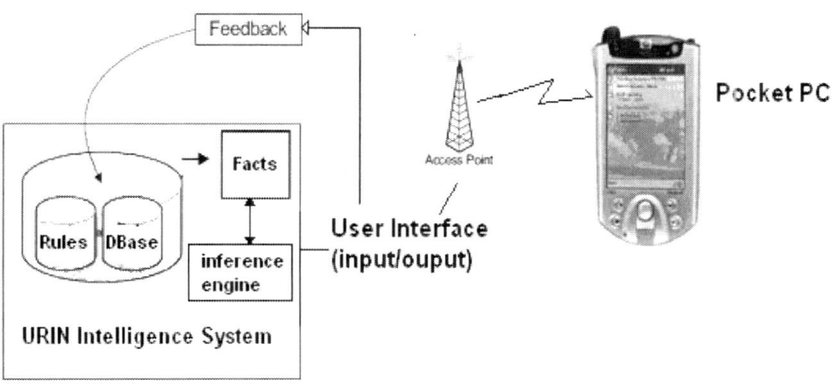

Figure 5. The intelligent system from a mobile pc or phone user, modified from [34].

CONCLUSION

The management of depression or other mental diseases is difficult but real occurrence [4]. The application of A.I. in clinical practice can be demonstrated beneficial as it could facilitate health professionals in taking critical and evidence-based medical decisions provided through fast and simply used mobile applications [32]. The most important advantage of the present approach is the understandable visibility of the systems' deep reasoning process from experts which can easily be modified according to their personal experience that additionally could be enriched with explanations about "why" each time the final decision was of that or the other type. The second is that according to the patient records that each time can be used the final system may "absorb" the specific approach of each group of experts' way of thinking, keeping scientific individuality intact.

Finally, future work could provide the user-friendly mobile version, written in other languages than English, of the system, with different stages of accessibility to be easily usable even from non-experts that could early detect abnormal behavior in the close community environment [34]. The usability of the system can intergrade some non-deep description of the reasoning in the text to give some general advice according to the final output to the non-experts expanding the range of well-educated patients away from multiple uncertified internet sources.

REFERENCES

[1] Weizmann-Henelius, G., Viemerö, V., & Eronen, M. (2004). Psychopathy in violent female offenders in Finland. *Psychopathology,* 37(5), 213-221.

[2] Achenbach, T. M., & Edelbrock, C. (1991). *Child behavior checklist.* Burlington (Vt), 7.

[3] Barton, C., Alexander, J. F., Waldron, H., Turner, C. W., & Warburton, J. (1985). Generalizing treatment effects of functional family therapy: Three replications. *The American Journal of Family Therapy,* 13(3), 16-26.

[4] American Psychiatric Association. (2013). *Diagnostic and statistical manual of mental disorders (DSM-5®).* American Psychiatric Pub.

[5] Beelmann, A., Pfingsten, U., & Lösel, F. (1994). Effects of training social competence in children: A meta-analysis of recent evaluation studies. *Journal of clinical child psychology,* 23(3), 260-271.

[6] Stumphauzer, J. S. (1976). Elimination of stealing by self-reinforcement of alternative behavior and family contracting. *Journal of Behavior Therapy and Experimental Psychiatry,* 7(3), 265-268.

[7] Lindberg, R. (2017). *Major Depressive Disorder and Marital Relationships.*

[8] Willner, P. (2017). The chronic mild stress (CMS) model of depression: History, evaluation and usage. *Neurobiology of Stress,* 6, 78-93.

[9] Diler, R. S., Goldstein, T. R., Hafeman, D., Merranko, J., Liao, F., Goldstein, B. I., ... & Keller, M. B. (2017). Distinguishing Bipolar Depression from Unipolar Depression in Youth: Preliminary Findings. *Journal of Child and Adolescent Psychopharmacology.*

[10] Maske, U. E., Hapke, U., Riedel-Heller, S. G., Busch, M. A., & Kessler, R. C. (2017). Respondents' report of a clinician-diagnosed depression in health surveys: comparison with DSM-IV mental disorders in the general adult population in Germany. *BMC psychiatry,* 17(1), 39.

[11] Harkness, A. R., Reynolds, S. M., & Lilienfeld, S. O. (2014). A review of systems for psychology and psychiatry: adaptive systems, personality psychopathology five (PSY–5), and the DSM–5. *Journal of personality assessment,* 96(2), 121-139.

[12] Kaklauskas, A. (2015). *Biometric and Intelligent Decision Making Support.* Springer.

[13] Naser, S. S. A., & Hamed, M. A. (2016). An Expert System for Mouth Problems in Infants and Children. *Journal of*

Multidisciplinary Engineering Science Studies (JMESS), 2(4), 468-476.

[14] Jackson, P. (1998). *Introduction to expert systems.*

[15] Nwigbo Stella, N., & Chuks, A. O. (2011). *Expert system: a catalyst in educational development in Nigeria.*

[16] Barzilay, R., McCullough, D., Rambow, O., DeCristofaro, J., Korelsky, T., & Lavoie, B. (1998). A new approach to expert system explanations. Cogentex Inc Ithaca NY.

[17] Sikchi, S. S., Sikchi, S., & Ali, M. S. (2013). Fuzzy expert systems (FES) for medical diagnosis. *International Journal of Computer Applications,* 63(11).

[18] Sandra, S. Depression: Questions You Have Answers You Need. *People's Medical Society* (1997). ISBN 978 1 882606 14 6.

[19] Judd, L. L., Schettler, P. J., Coryell, W., Akiskal, H. S., & Fiedorowicz, J. G. (2013). Overt irritability/anger in unipolar major depressive episodes: past and current characteristics and implications for long-term course. *JAMA psychiatry,* 70(11), 1171-1180.

[20] Qin, P. (2003). The relationship of suicide risk to family history of suicide and psychiatric disorders. *Psychiatric Times,* 20(13), 62-62.

[21] Pillemer, K., Suitor, J. J., Pardo, S., & Henderson, C. (2010). Mothers' differentiation and depressive symptoms among adult children. *Journal of Marriage and Family,* 72(2), 333-345.

[22] Coiera, E. (1997). *Guide to medical informatics, the internet and telemedicine.* Chapman & Hall, Ltd.

[23] Duda, R. O., & Shortliffe, E. H. (1983). Expert systems research. *Science,* 220 (4594), 261-268.

[24] Liao, S. H. (2005). Expert system methodologies and applications—a decade review from 1995 to 2004. *Expert systems with applications,* 28(1), 93-103.

[25] Archer, R. P., Handel, R. W., Ben-Porath, Y. S., & Tellegen, A. (2016). Minnesota Multiphasic Personality Inventory-Adolescent-Restructured Form (MMPI-A-RF): Administration, scoring, interpretation, and technical manual.

[26] Almurshidi, S. H., & Naser, S. S. A. (2017). *Stomach Disease Intelligent Tutoring System.*

[27] Naser, S. S. A., & Alhabbash, M. I. (2016). Male Infertility Expert system Diagnoses and Treatment. *American Journal of Innovative Research and Applied Sciences,* 2(4).

[28] Edition, F., & American Psychiatric Association. (1994). *Diagnostic and statistical manual of mental disorders.* Washington, American Psychological Association.

[29] Koutsojannis C, Nabil EA, Tsimara M, Hatzilygeroudis I. (2009). Using machine learning techniques to improve the behavior of a medical decision support system for prostate diseases, Intelligent Systems Design and Applications, 2009. ISDA'09. Pisa, Italy Nov. 30, 2009 to Dec. 2, 2009, pp: 341-346.

[30] Schnyer DM, Clasen PC, Gonzalez C, Beevers CG. (2017). Evaluating the diagnostic utility of applying a machine-learning algorithm to diffusion tensor MRI measures in individuals with major depressive disorder. *Psychiatry Res Neuroimaging.* 2017 Jun 30;264:1-9.

[31] Koutsojannis C, Lithari C, Hatzilygeroudis I. Managing urinary incontinence through hand-held real-time decision support aid. *Computer methods and programs in biomedicine* 03/2012; 107(1):84-9.

[32] https://www.technologyreview.com/s/603200/voice-analysis-tech-could-diagnose-disease/.

[33] https://www.vox.com/science-and-health/2017/4/4/15073652/precision-psychiatry-depression.

[34] http://x2ai.com/.

BIOGRAPHICAL SKETCHES

Andreas Andrikopoulos

Dr Andreas Andrikopoulos (male) elaborated his PhD thesis in School of Medicine, Lab of Medical Physics in Democritus University of Thrace, Greece. His PhD thesis is about restriction of radiofrequency exposure from microwave diathermy units based on distribution simulation upon radiation interactions. From 2014 till now he started to instruct as an Associate Professor at the Department of Optics and Optometry at University of Patras, Greece. He is also employed as a laboratory collaborator of Researching Laboratory of Health Physics & Computational Intelligence (University of Patras) with clinical experience in measurements and prevention issues of electromagnetic radiation since 2008. His research interests include: medical informatics, health-physics, non-ionizing radiation protection, radiation sickness and genetic damage, mechanisms of electromagnetic interaction with living tissue, occupational radiation exposure, electromagnetic hypersensitivity, mobile phone radiation and health risks.

Constantinos Koutsojannis

Associate Professor, Constantinos Koutsojannis is currently Director of Laboratory of Health Physics & Computational Intelligence, in University of Patras. He is Medical Physicist and expert in Medical Informatics. He is teaching Biophysics, Biostatistics, Research Methodology, Computational Intelligence, Artificial Intelligence and Medical Informatics in several undergraduate and master programs of University of Patras, University of Ioannina and University of Athens. He is involved in a number of Research and Development National and European Projects concerning Artificial Intelligence and serves as a consultant in Artificial Intelligence Working Group as well as full member of Project Committee of European Federation of Medical Physics. His research deals with Biophysics and Medical Applications with Artificial

Intelligence on diagnosis, treatment and training using methods of Medical Knowledge representation and extraction from patient data record, medical textbooks and field experts. He has published in a number international journals, conferences and books on the fields of his interest.

Ioannis Hatzilygeroudis

Dr. Ioannis Hatzilygeroudis is Professor in the Department of Computer Engineering & Informatics of the University of Patras. He is Associate Editor-in-Chief of the International Journal of Artificial Intelligence Tools (IJAIT). He has also been a member of Program Committees in over 70 international conferences and has organized several invited / special sessions in international conferences. He has published more than 100 scientific papers in international journals, volumes and conference proceedings. He has also participated in a number of National and European projects both as a partner and as a coordinator. She has been teaching programming for over 15 years. His main research interests are: Artificial Intelligence, Knowledge Representation, Knowledge Based / Experienced Systems, Intelligent Educational Systems and Intelligent E-Learning.

In: Medical Knowledge Extraction ...
Editor: C. M. Koutsojannis
ISBN: 978-1-53617-925-5

Chapter 8

A Hybrid Intelligent System for Diagnosis of Male Impotence with the Use of Direct Knowledge Representation

Constantinos Koutsojannis*[1,*]*, Grigorios Beligiannis*[2]*,
***Perimenis Petros*[3] *and Ioannis Hatzilygeroudis*[4]**
[1]Laboratory of Health Physics & Computational Intelligence,
University of Patras, Patras, Greece
[2]Department of Farm Organization and Management,
School of Natural Resources and Enterprise Management,
University of Patras, Agrinio, Greece
[3]Department of Urology, University of Patras, Patras, Greece
[4]Computer Engineering & Informatics Department University of Patras,
Patras, Greece

* Corresponding Author's Email: ckoutsog1@gmail.com.

Abstract

Manipulation of male sexual dysfunction (or impotence) that concerns 10% of the male population requires expertise and a great experience. Different diagnostic approaches according to medical as well as psychosocial and cultural characteristics of patients are usually followed. Additionally, the traditional health care model of a resident doctor interacting with a senior staff doctor in a mentoring role is not possible in today's world of expert shortages and high patient loads. In this contribution, an intelligent medical Hybrid Decision Support System (HDSS) for diagnosis of male impotence is proposed, in order to assist novice doctors in making sound clinical judgments. The diagnosis process, the linguistic variables, and their values are modeled using a fuzzy expert system (FESMI) module based on expert knowledge, statistical analysis of patients' records taken from a hospital database and the existing literature. To overcome the limitations of knowledge representation and difficulties of fuzzy computing, genetic algorithms were additionally used to evolve rules from the same database. Both modules – fuzzy and genetic – produce in parallel their own diagnosis and an associated reliability value. The latter is a function of the "sensitivity" and "specificity" of the result based on the input-output parameters of a training data set. These typical values are represented by fuzzy sets and accordingly the degree to which each diagnosis satisfies the true condition of the respective patient is computed. The overall diagnosis reliability is obtained by considering the conjunction of this constraint satisfaction (i.e., the maximum of the individual reliability values). Experimental results show that the proposed system performs quite better compared to the pure Fuzzy Expert System and about 90%, as well as the expert, did. Finally, the use of a hybrid model integrating two different Cognitive Computing technologies, such as Fuzzy Logic and Genetic Algorithms, resulted in reducing the knowledge elicitation, speeding up the model choice process, and as far as knowledge modeling is concerned, better coding of human reasoning.

Keywords: fuzzy expert system, medical decision support, hybrid model, genetic algorithms, evolutionary computing, male impotence

INTRODUCTION

Human sexual dysfunction (or impotence) is characterized by disturbances in sexual desire and in psychophysiological changes associated with the sexual response cycle in men and women. There are three types of sexual dysfunction found in men: erectile dysfunction, premature ejaculation, and a low sexual desire. An estimated 10% of the male population experience chronic erectile dysfunction (ED), however as few as 5% of them seek treatment. ED may affect 50% of men between the ages of 40 and 70 [23, 23a]. Furthermore, the transient lost or inadequate erection may affect men of all ages. Most men experience this inability at some stage in their lives, usually by the age of 40, but are not psychologically affected by it. It has many causes, most of which are treatable. It is not an inevitable consequence of aging. Due to experts in this field, more men seek help and return to normal sexual activity because of improved, successful treatments for ED. Causes of ED can be both psychological and/or organic [31], [32]. Manipulation of the dysfunction requires expertise and a great experience. Doctors, even urologists, cannot usually perform a typical evaluation and propose a treatment strategy. Different approaches according to medical as well as psychosocial and cultural characteristics of patients should be usually followed. Specification of the parameters and their possible impacts on the diagnosis and treatment are still under consideration and vogue. So, the creation of an intelligent system to assist non-expert doctors in making an initial diagnosis is quite desirable.

"Soft Computing" is a term that represents a number of intelligent techniques, such as fuzzy logic (FL), neural computing (NC), evolutionary computation (EC), machine learning (ML) and probabilistic reasoning (PR) [22]. Although soft computing techniques are by themselves successfully used in solving many problems, this is not always the case, especially in complex domains, where problems are ill-defined. It is evident that hybrid intelligent systems (HISs) have been more and more used to solve problems in such domains, like industry, medicine [12] and finance [35]. A HIS is a system that combines more than one soft computing or other (e.g., hard computing) intelligent technique [25] for solving problems in a way that produces better results than if each component technique were used by itself. There are various combinations of intelligent techniques used in medical systems (for a detailed account see [11]) that cover many medical areas (Cardiology, Radiology, Neurology, Cytology, Nuclear medicine, Dermatology, Gynaecology, Oncology, Surgery, etc). One of them is the combination of FL and genetic algorithms (GAs), a type of EC. There are only a few systems that use this combination. For example, in [33] GAs are used to solve logical equations in a medical diagnostic system. Also, an EC based fuzzy inference system is used to assess brain-gut interaction in [38]. Finally, the system presented in [8] combines NC, FL and a GA. However, GA is used to optimize the hidden layer of a neural network.

In this paper, we present a Hybrid Intelligent System for diagnosis of Male Impotence (HISMI), which combines a fuzzy expert system with a genetic algorithm-driven rule-based system. The fuzzy expert system, called FESMI (Fuzzy Expert System for Male Impotence), is a revised version of an initial effort reported in [24]. The genetic algorithm-driven rule-based intelligent system (GADIS) is a more complete version of the one reported in [17]. GADIS is a similar effort to [36]. HISMI goes beyond those efforts by combining FESMI and GADIS to make diagnoses for male impotence. The choice of which of them is activated depends on the user query. We are not aware of any other similar attempt applied to a medical domain. The paper is organized as follows: in section 1 we introduce impotence, in section 2 we briefly introduce fuzzy logic and evolutionary computing as parts of cognitive computing field and the expert's diagnostic and therapeutic model, in sections 3 and 4 we describe our system and some aspects of its implementation issues, in section 5 we present our evaluation results from real patient data, in section 6 we discuss our results due to the hybrid modeling approach and finally in the last section we conclude.

FUZZY LOGIC AND FUZZY EXPERT SYSTEMS

In real world, people usually make decisions and solve problems by using imprecise rather than precise knowledge. Fuzzy Logic (FL), originally introduced by Lofti Zadeh in 1965 [42], resembles human reasoning in making decisions and solve problems based on imprecise or approximate knowledge. FL was introduced as an alternative problem-solving methodology, which is a generalization of classical Boolean logic. FL uses linguistic variables representing a continuous range of truth values and allows for intermediate truth values, i.e., values between the two values (0, 1) of the conventional binary logic. It can be considered as a superset of Boolean or crisp logic. FL is based on fuzzy set theory [43]. Linguistic variables are represented by fuzzy sets. In this way, FL can represent uncertainty and vagueness and provides formalized tools for dealing with imprecision.

So, FL gives us a language, with formal syntax and semantics, in which we can translate qualitative knowledge about the problem to be solved. In particular, FL allows us to use linguistic variables (e.g., age, smoking) to model knowledge. These variables take fuzzy values that are characterized by linguistic terms (e.g., low-medium-high or yes-no). Each fuzzy value corresponds to a fuzzy set, which is a mapping between crisp values and membership values. They have overlapping domains.

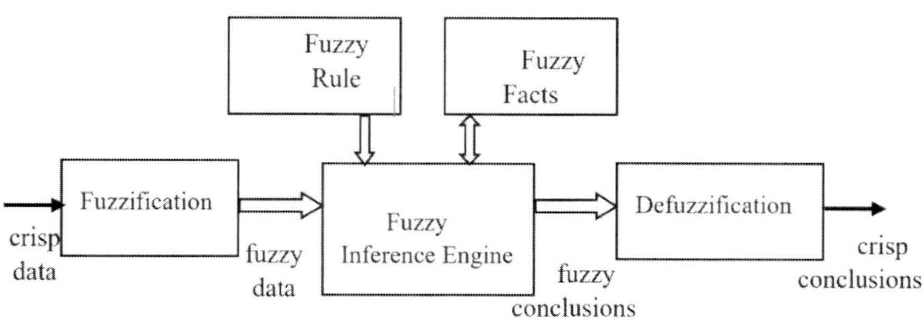

Figure 1. Structure of and process in a Fuzzy Expert System.

A practical form of FL is fuzzy rules. Fuzzy rules are of two types, Mamdani and Sugeno. Mamdani type rules are best suited for diagnostic problems. They have the form "if x is A and y is B then z is C", where x, y, z are fuzzy (linguistic) variables and A, B, C are fuzzy (linguistic) values. Reasoning with fuzzy rules is based on a generalized modus-ponens rule, which gives robustness with respect to variations in the system parameters, disturbances, etc.

An expert system (ES) is a system that resembles human expert reasoning and usually uses production rules to represent knowledge. Using fuzzy rules instead makes it a fuzzy expert system (FES). An FES has a somewhat different structure and inference flow than a conventional ES. A typical fuzzy expert system consists of a rule base, corresponding membership functions and an inference procedure (Figure 1). An important thing is that fuzzy rules retain the naturalness of conventional rules, at least a syntax level. Compared to classical ESs, FESs can handle non-linear relations between inputs and outputs.

Reasoning in an FES includes three stages: fuzzification, inference, defuzzification. In fuzzification, the crisp input values (from the user) are converted to membership degrees, by applying the corresponding membership functions that become the truth degrees of the corresponding conditions of the fuzzy rules. In the inference stage, first, the degrees of the conditions of the fuzzy rules are combined to produce the degrees of the truth of the conclusions. The MIN method is used here. According to that, the degree of truth of a conclusion is the minimum of the degrees of the conditions of the corresponding rule (AND fuzzy operation) and its membership function is clipped off at a height corresponding to that minimum. Afterward, all the degrees assigned to the same conclusions (i.e., rule outputs) are combined into a single degree using the MAX method. According to that, the combined output degree of truth is the maximum of the degrees (OR fuzzy operation) and its membership function is clipped off at a height corresponding to that maximum. Finally, the clipped off membership functions of all outputs are aggregated to form the combined fuzzy output. In defuzzification, the fuzzy output is converted to a crisp value. Here, the well-known centroid method is used.

According to that method, the crisp output value is the x-coordinate value of the center of gravity of the aggregate membership function [29].

It is well known that medical knowledge is often characterized by inaccuracy. Medical terms do not usually have a clear-cut interpretation. Thus, FL makes it possible to define inexact medical entities via fuzzy sets. The final model is empirically-based, relying on the expert's experience rather than their technical understanding of the system. Fuzzy rules are used to describe the desired system response in terms of linguistic variables rather than mathematical formulas. Thus is ideal for medical complex problems, where knowledge modeling cannot easily be abstracted.

During the last decade, a number of fuzzy techniques have been introduced that have been extensively applied to medical systems [1, 24, 9, 4]. The basic reason is that fuzzy logic provides reasoning methods for approximate inference, that is, inference with inaccurate (or fuzzy) terms. Evolutionary computation (EC) techniques have been developed by attempting to imitate the mechanisms of natural selection and natural genetics. They have been around for quite some time, but have recently gained popularity, due to the advances in computing equipment, which make their implementation feasible and efficient. One of the most popular approaches to evolutionary computation is Genetic Algorithms (GAs), initially introduced by John H. Holland [20]. GAs operate on binary string structures, analogous to biological creatures. These structures are evolving in time according to the rule of survival of the fittest by using a randomized, yet structured information exchange scheme. Thus, in every generation, a new set of binary strings is created, using parts of the fittest members of the old set [18, 27].

GAs process a binary coding of the parameter space and work on it. This coding (which is an essential part of the GA design procedure) results in the formation of binary strings. Having decided on the binary coding to be used, an initial set of strings (a population) is created at random. Next, a set of operators is applied to this initial population to generate successive generations that hopefully will improve over time. An objective function (usually referred to as fitness function in GA terminology) serves as a measure of goodness of a string. Several operators have been proposed at times; however, three simple operators perform well in a wide variety of search and optimization problems. These are the *selection* operator, the *crossover* operator and the *mutation* operator [28, 37].

Selection is a process by virtue of which individual strings are tentatively selected as candidate parents for the next generation, according to their objective function values. The selection is performed by a randomized technique ensuring the survival of the fittest; its details may vary according to the specific problem that the GA is designed for, but a biased roulette wheel selection scheme usually suffices. Once a string is selected, an exact replica of itself is made and entered into a mating pool to be tentatively used as a parent of the next generation.

Crossover is the process by virtue of which the actual mating is performed. Again, several methods of crossing over have been proposed at times, each having its relative merits. The common feature of all crossover operators is that they select (randomly) pairs of mates out of the tentative population generated by the reproduction operator and they create new individuals (binary strings) with hopefully improved fitness.

The mutation is the occasional (with a small probability) random alteration of the value of a strong position. By itself, the mutation is a random walk through the coded parameter space. It is usually used sparingly, together with the two previously mentioned operators, in order to ensure that important information contained within strings may not be prematurely lost.

Genetic Algorithms

Evolutionary computation (EC) techniques have been developed by attempting to imitate the mechanisms of natural selection and natural genetics. They have been around for quite some time, but have recently gained popularity, due to the advances in computing equipment, which make their implementation feasible and efficient. One of the most popular approaches to evolutionary computation is Genetic Algorithms (GAs), initially introduced by John H. Holland [20]. GAs operate on binary string structures, analogous to biological creatures. These structures are evolving in time according to the rule of survival of the fittest by using a randomized, yet structured information exchange scheme. Thus, in every generation, a new set of binary strings is created, using parts of the fittest members of the old set [18, 27].

GAs process a binary coding of the parameter space and work on it. This coding (which is an essential part of the GA design procedure) results in the formation of binary strings. Having decided on the binary coding to be used, an initial set of strings (a population) is created at random. Next, a set of operators is applied to this initial population to generate successive generations that hopefully will improve over time. An objective function (usually referred to as fitness function in GA terminology) serves as a measure of goodness of a string. Several operators have been proposed at times; however, three simple operators perform well in a wide variety of search and optimization problems. These are the *selection* operator, the *crossover* operator and the *mutation* operator [28, 37].

Selection is a process by virtue of which individual strings are tentatively selected as candidate parents for the next generation, according to their objective function values. The selection is performed by a randomized technique ensuring the survival of the fittest; its details may vary according to the specific problem that the GA is designed for, but a biased roulette wheel selection scheme usually suffices. Once a string is selected, an exact replica of itself is made and entered into a mating pool to be tentatively used as a parent of the next generation.

Crossover is the process by virtue of which the actual mating is performed. Again, several methods of crossing over have been proposed at times, each having its relative merits. The common feature of all crossover operators is that they select (randomly) pairs of mates out of the tentative population generated by the reproduction operator and they create new individuals (binary strings) with hopefully improved fitness.

The mutation is the occasional (with a small probability) random alteration of the value of a string position. By itself, the mutation is a random walk through the coded parameter space. It is usually used sparingly, together with the two previously mentioned operators, in order to ensure that important information contained within strings may not be prematurely lost.

It should be noted that several other (more advanced) operators, as well as different reproductive schemes, have been proposed at times. However, the three operators presented in the previous paragraphs have been proved [39, 40, 14], to be both computationally simple and effective in attacking a wide number of important search and optimization problems.

In Figure 2, the basic cycle of the GA we use in this paper is presented. At the start, an initial population is generated based on the selected representation. Afterward, the members of the population are evaluated based on an objective function and the training data set. The objective function evaluates how good is each member of the population, based on how many entries of the data set it matches. After that, if the termination criterion (e.g., the number of generations set) is met the process stops and the best individual (i.e., that with the maximum objective value) is selected as the solution. If not, three operators (selection, crossover, and mutation) are applied to the population and a new population is generated. Again, the objective function is used to evaluate its members and so on.

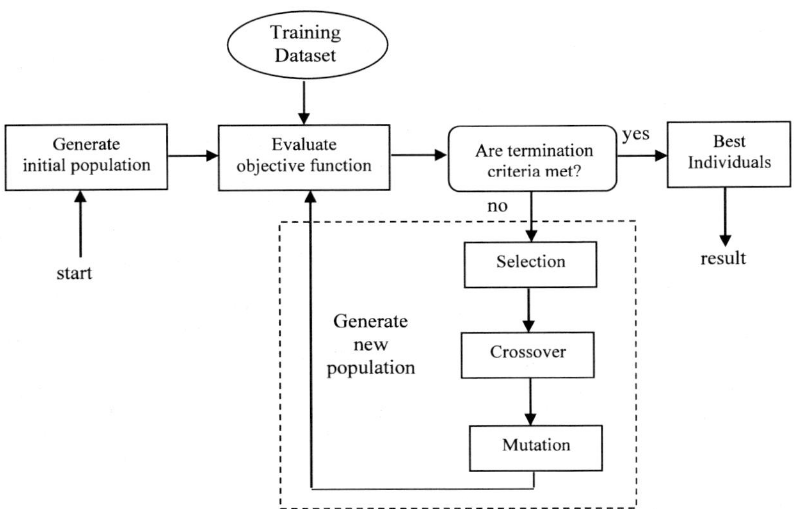

Figure 2. A Simple Genetic Algorithm.

Medical Knowledge Modelling

The knowledge modeling (KM) task consists in extracting knowledge mainly from the domain experts and constructing a model of how diagnoses are performed.

An appropriate diagnosis of ED requires urology doctors with long experience in Andrology. One of the problems is that there is not any widely accepted approach yet. Therefore, except for the fact that we had a number of interviews with an expert in the field, we also used patient records and bibliographical sources. Our approach to knowledge modeling included three steps. First, we constructed an abstract model of the basic diagnosis process, where we specified patient data entities that play a role in diagnoses, either intermediate or final. We relied on the expert and the literature at this step. Then, we specified the parameters that play a role in each entity of the process model. At this step, we relied on the expert and the patient records. Finally, we determined the relations between parameters and intermediate and final diagnoses. We had, however, to iterate a number of times to tune the model.

Medical Diagnosis Process Modelling

We constructed the model of Figure 3 for the diagnosis and treatment process of ED. In Figure 3, the vertical bold lines indicate inference nodes. According to that, initially, an urologist-andrologist requires the following information [31, 32]: (a) medical history, (b) psychosocial history, (c) sexual history, (d) physical examination and (e) some diagnostic tests, which can be characterized as obligatory. At this stage, based on them, an initial diagnosis is made, concerning the nature of the cause of the problem. There are two possible initial diagnoses: the cause of the problem is (a) possibly psychogenic or (b) possibly organic.

To confirm and/or further specialize the initial diagnosis, the expert requires further information related to diagnostic laboratory tests that could be characterized as advanced. Once the expert gets results of them, they may give a final diagnosis, which can be one of (a) *endocrinopathy* or (b) *neuropathy*. However, to be able to handle the spectrum of all possible diagnoses, the expert needs some specialized tests too. Given them, the expert can make the final diagnosis, which can be, apart from the above two, one of (c) *arteriopathy*, (d) *venooclusive insufficiency* and (e) psychogenic. This makes the diagnosis process quite complicated. For example, although an initial diagnosis for 'possibly psychogenic' may be made, it may turn out that the final diagnosis is 'arteriopathy' or '*venooclusive insufficiency*', i.e., a type of organic cause, due to results of specialized tests.

Given the complexity of the diagnosis model of Figure 3 and the cost of the advanced and specialized tests, the question that naturally arises is whether we can make a quite realistic diagnosis based only on the patient data related to the first five categories of patient data above. This would save time and reduce the cost of diagnosis. This simplified model is depicted in Figure 4, which is actually a model that is used in countries or in cases where advanced and specialized tests are not available or too expensive. The problem with this model is that the relations between patient data parameters and final diagnoses are difficult to acquire from bibliographical sources or even experts.

DIAGNOSIS PARAMETERS

Based on our expert urologists, we specified a set of parameters for each of the entities in the process model that represent patient data (Figure 3) that play a role in diagnosis. We also used a statistical analysis method (Pearson analysis) to evaluate which of the parameters recorded in the patient records are significant for the intermediate and final diagnosis. We analyzed about 420 patient records from the patient database of the "Andrology Laboratory" of the Department of Urology of the University Hospital of Patras, Greece. We found that parameters like chronology, alcohol, and weight are significant, although they were underestimated by the experts. Finally, we resulted in the 22 parameters presented in Figure 5.

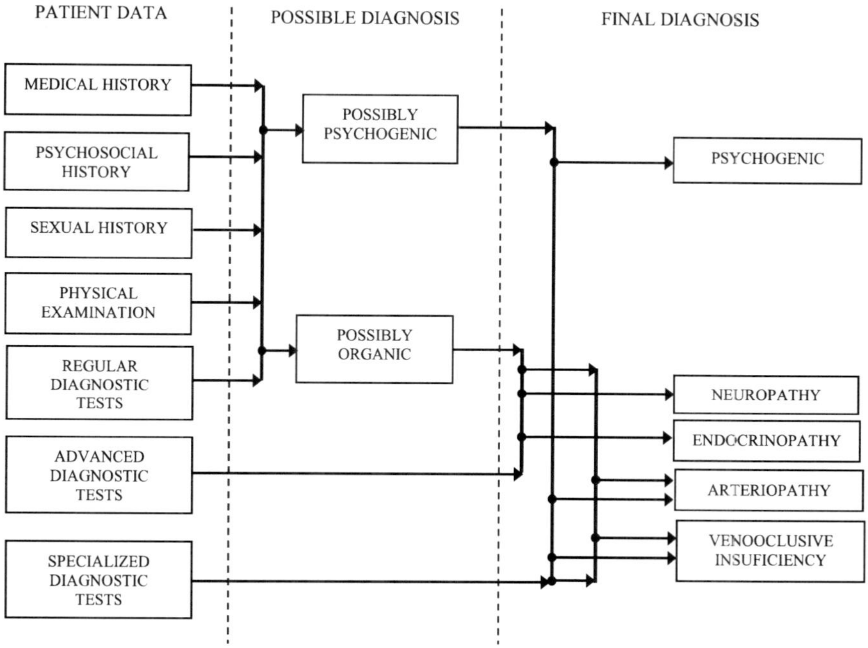

Figure 3. ED Diagnosis Process Model.

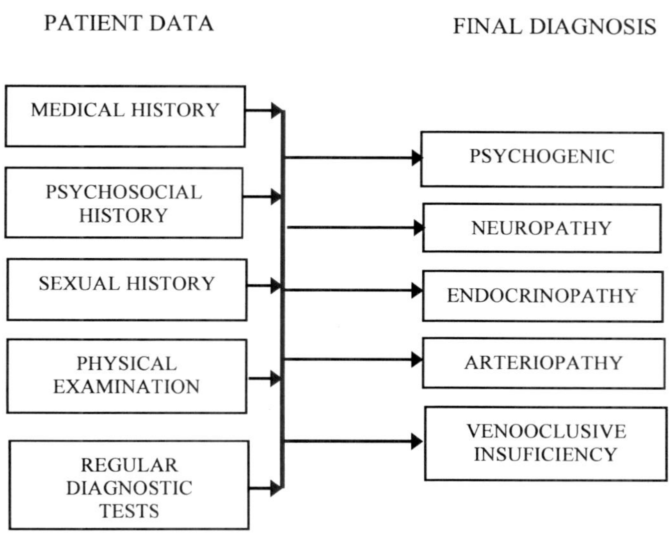

Figure 4. ED Simplified Diagnosis Process Model.

Medical history	Psychosocial history	Advanced tests
• *onset* • *non-coital erection* • *onanism* • *diabetes mellitus* • *coronary artery* • *prostate* • *neuropathies* Sexual history • *chronolgy*	• *age* • *depression* • *smoking* • *alcohol* Physical examination • *blood pressure* • *weight* Regular tests • *blood sugar* • *cholesterol*	• *neurophysiological* • *hormonal evaluation* Specialized tests • *NPT* • *PIP* • *Doppler* • *DICC*

Figure 5. Input Parameters.

According to the model, we distinguish between input, intermediate and final parameters.

- Input parameters:
  - All parameters of Figure 5 (their values vary).
- Intermediate parameters:
  - *possible diagnosis* (values: psychogenic, organic)
- Output parameters:
  - *final diagnosis* (values: psychogenic, arteriopathy, venooclusive insufficiency, neuropathy, endocrinopathy)

The dependencies among parameters are shown in Tables 1a and 1b.

FUZZY EXPERT SYSTEM FOR MALE IMPOTENCE (FESMI)

In this section, we present a fuzzy expert system is called FESMI that used to implement the Diagnosis Process Model. FESMI has the structure of Figure 1, which is similar to the typical structure of such systems [30]. The knowledge base of the expert system includes fuzzy rules, which are symbolic (if-then) rules with linguistic variables (e.g., age). Linguistic variables take linguistic values (e.g., young, middle-aged, old). Each linguistic value is represented by a fuzzy set: a range of crisp (i.e., non-linguistic) values with different degrees of membership to the set. The degrees are specified via a membership function. The variables of the conditions (or antecedents) of a rule are inputs and the variable of its conclusion (or consequent) the output of the system.

Table 1a. Input-intermediate parameter dependences

Input/Intermediate	Possibly Psychogenic	Possibly Organic
onset	X	
non-coital erection	X	
onanism	X	
diabetes mellitus		X
coronary artery		X
prostate	X	
neuropathies		X
chronology	X	X
age	X	X
depression	X	
smoking	X	X
alcohol		X
blood pressure		X
weight		X
hormonal evaluation		X
cholesterol		X

Table 1b. Intermediate-output parameter dependences

Intermediate/ Output	Psychogenic	Venooclusive insufficiency	Artieriopathy	Neuropathy	Endocrinopathy
possible diagnosis	X	X	X	X	X
NPT	X	X	X		
PIP	X	X	X		
Doppler	X	X	X		
DICC	X	X	X		
Neurophy-siologic test	X	X	X	X	

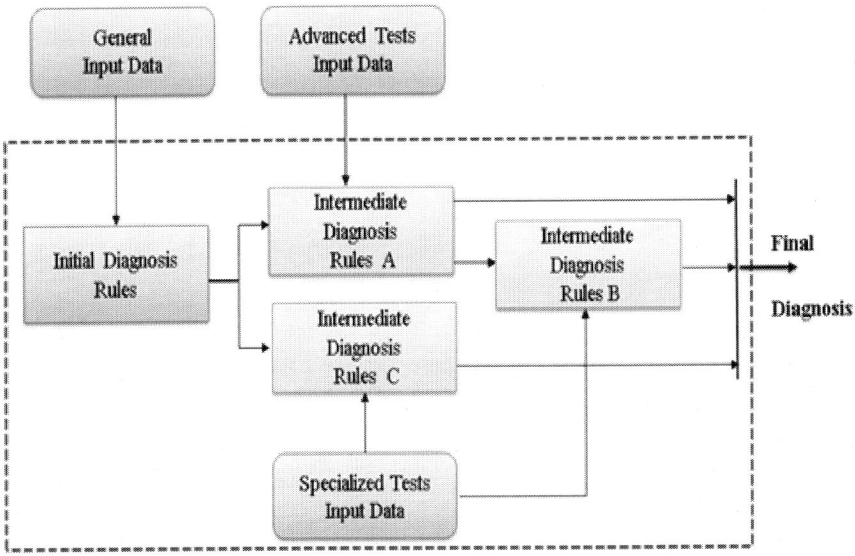

Figure 6. Inference Flow in FESMI.

To reflect the process model of Figure 3, we organized fuzzy rules in four groups: Initial Diagnosis Rules, Intermediate Diagnosis Rules A, Intermediate Diagnosis Rules B and Intermediate Diagnosis Rules C. The current patient data can be stored in the Database as facts. Each time the reasoning process requires a value, it gets it from the database. Patient data can be also given by the user, in an interactive mode. Figure 6 presents how the rule groups and the facts/user are used/participates during the reasoning process to simulate the diagnosis process.

Initial diagnosis rules result in an initial (possible) diagnosis (one of 'possibly psychogenic' or 'possibly organic') based on the 'General Input Data', which are data (values) for the parameters related to the parameters of 'medical history', 'psychosocial history', 'sexual history', 'physical examination' and 'regular diagnostic tests'. Intermediate diagnosis rules A are employed in case that the initial diagnosis is 'possibly psychogenic' and based on 'Specialized Tests Input Data' result in a final diagnosis (one of 'psychogenic', 'arteriopathy' and 'venooclusive insufficiency'). Intermediate diagnosis rules B are employed in case that the initial diagnosis is 'possibly organic' and based on 'Advanced Tests Input Data' result either in a final diagnosis (one of 'endocrinopathy' or 'neuropathy') or in an intermediate diagnosis, which focus on the group of 'arteriopathy' and 'venooclusive insufficiency'. Intermediate diagnosis rules C are employed in the latter case and based on 'Specialized Tests Input Data' decide on 'arteriopathy' or 'venooclusive insufficiency' as the final diagnosis.

IMPLEMENTATION ISSUES

Linguistic values and corresponding membership functions have been determined by the aid of the experts, the statistical analysis of patient data and the literature. Examples of values and corresponding membership functions are shown in Figure 7 and Figure 8.

The system has been developed in FuzzyCLIPS 6.1b [21] expert system shell. Finally, about 93 fuzzy rules have been constructed. Patient data in the Database are organized by using FuzzyCLIPS templates. For example, the following rule:

Rule 3: If ***onset*** *is acute and* ***non-coital*** *is yes and* ***onanism*** *is yes and* ***chronology*** *is recent and* ***age*** *is middleage and* ***smoking*** *is high then* ***psychogenic*** *is very high*

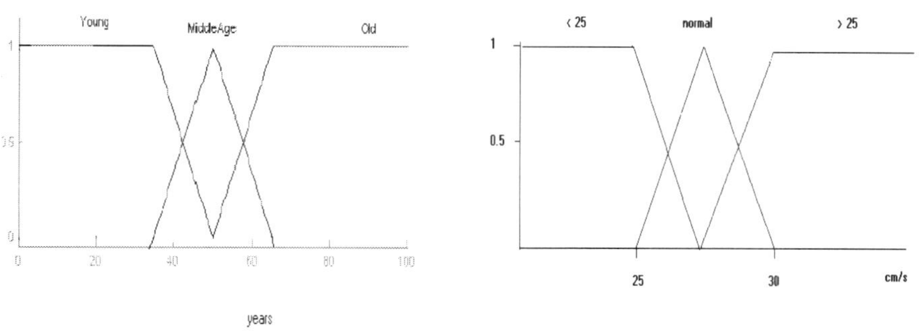

Figure 7. Linguistic values and membership functions of 'age' and 'doppler_test'.

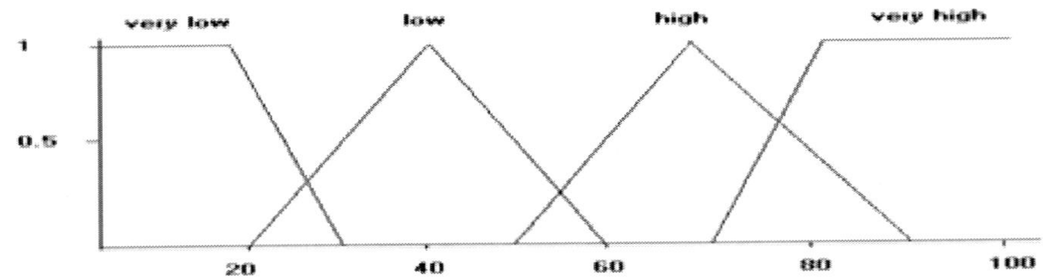

Figure 8. Linguistic values and membership function of 'psychogenic_diagnosis'.

To implement reasoning flow, different priorities have been assigned to different rule groups. For example, priority of the rules in 'Initial Diagnosis Rules' group is greater than that of the rules in 'Intermediate Diagnosis Rules A' and 'Intermediate Diagnosis Rules B' groups and priority of the rules in 'Intermediate Diagnosis Rules A' group is greater than that of rules in 'Intermediate Diagnosis Rules B'. This assures that rules in 'Initial Diagnosis Rules' group will be examined before those in 'Intermediate Diagnosis Rules A' and 'Intermediate Diagnosis Rules B' groups and rules in 'Intermediate Diagnosis Rules A' group will be examined before those in 'Intermediate Diagnosis Rules B' in the inference flow.

Genetic Algorithm Driven Intelligent System (GADIS)

To implement the simplified model of Figure 4, we created GADIS, a Genetic Algorithm Driven Intelligent System. Given the difficulty of acquiring knowledge from bibliographical sources or experts, we are using two genetic algorithms to extract symbolic rules from available medical data. In this section, we present the basic aspects of GADIS.

The architecture of GADIS is depicted in Figure 9. It consists of the following units: user interface (UI), classifiers producing genetic algorithm (CPGA), rule extracting genetic algorithm (REGA), medical database (MDB), rule base (RB) and inference engine (IE). Actually, RB and IE constitute the run-time system. CPGA, REGA and MDB are used off-line.

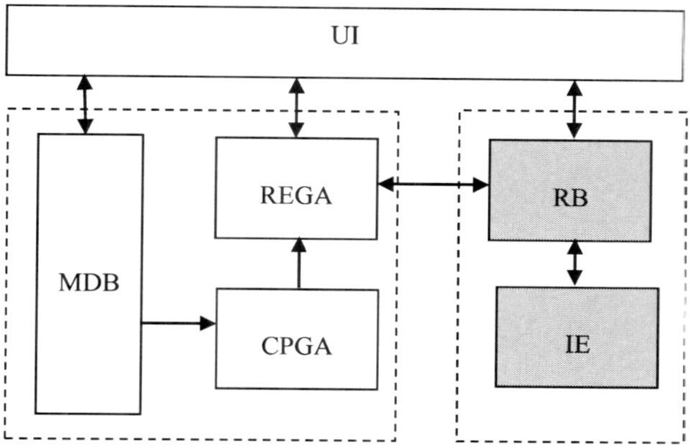

Figure 9. GADIS Architecture.

MDB contains patient data organized in groups. Each group refers to one of the possible diagnoses that the system can make (psychogenic, arteriopathy, venooclusive insufficiency, neuropathy, endocrinopathy). In the off-line mode, CPGA is successively applied to the data from each group in the MDB and produces a diagnosis classifier for each data group. The classifiers are then used by REGA to produce the evolved rules, which are then suitably transformed and update the RB. UI is the means for user communication and interference with the system, where and when it is necessary.

The rule base evolution process is depicted in Figure 10. From the available medical data, 60% from each diagnosis group is used as a training set, while the remaining 40% is left to be used as a test set.

The system creates the initial population of the GA, based on binary strings, and triggers the GA evolution process. After a few generations, the GA provides five different binary strings each corresponding to one of the five different possible diagnoses (psychogenic, arteriopathy, endocrinopathy, venooclusive insufficiency, and neuropathy). Each binary string constitutes a diagnosis classifier pattern for the corresponding diagnosis category.

Each such diagnosis classifier comprises a binary string that matches most of the provided training data of a specific diagnosis category. In this way, each diagnosis classifier contains the necessary information required by a rule that would correctly classify most of the provided training data. After that, the rule extraction procedure is taking over. Based on the characteristics of the five different diagnosis classifiers, this procedure results in a set of five different production rules each corresponding to a different diagnosis category. After the extraction of the rules is completed, the rule base is updated. We use the term 'updated' and not the term 'created', because this off-line process can be periodically repeated, given that adequate new patient data has been added to MDB.

GAs, in general, operate on binary string structures, analogous to biological creatures (genomes). These structures are evolving in time according to the rule of survival of the fittest, by using a randomized, yet structured, information exchange scheme. Thus, in every generation, a new set of binary strings is created, using parts of the fittest members of the old set. GAs process a binary coding of the parameter space and work on it. This coding (which is an essential part of the GA design procedure) results in the formation of binary strings.

In our case, the coding scheme comprises the 22 parameters, specified in Section 4.2, that represent the factors which diagnosis of male impotence is based on. Each parameter is coded into a binary string. This binary string is, in fact, the genome of the GA that will be evolved. Each parameter is coded using a 31-bits binary string. For example, parameter 'age', which can take nine different values (denoted by the from 1 to 9), is coded into the binary strings

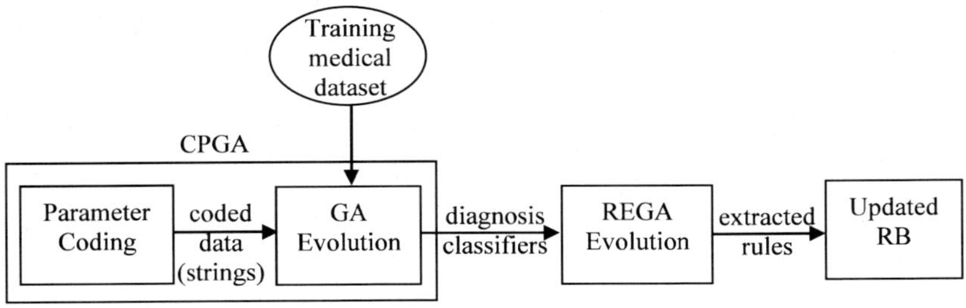

Figure 10. GA Based Rule Evolution Process.

$$\underbrace{000...000}_{27}0001 \quad \text{to} \quad \underbrace{000...000}_{27}1001$$

respectively (actually only the four last digits are required, the rest are used because of the implementation tool-see Section 6.6). On the other hand, parameter 'prostate', which is a yes-no (denoted by the integers 1 and 2) parameter, is coded into the binary strings

$$\underbrace{000...000}_{27}0001 \quad \text{and} \quad \underbrace{000...000}_{27}0010$$

respectively. Each binary string constitutes a gene of the genome of the GA. As a result, the whole genome length equals 682 (= 22 x 31) bits (Figure 10). A set of such genomes constitutes the GA's population.

$$\underbrace{\underbrace{0000..0011}_{31} \ \ldots \ \underbrace{0000..1100}_{31}}_{22}$$

Figure 11. The structure of the genome used in the evolution procedure of the GA used for creating diagnosis classifiers.

```
for i = 1 to m do
    fitness = 0;
    for j = 1 to 22 do
      for k =1 to n do
        if g[i, j] = d[k, j]
          then matches = matches+1;
        endif
      endfor
      if matches >= limit
        then fitness =fitness + 1;
      endif
    endfor
endfor
```

Figure 12. Algorithm for fitness computation.

The steps of the GA, which is a classical one, are presented in Figure 2. The initial population is generated using a set of random binary strings created by the parameter coding unit.

This process is repeated for each different diagnosis category. The termination criterion is the number of generations, that is the evolution process is terminated when a specific number of generations (in our case 5) are completed. While the termination criterion is not met, the whole evolution process is taking place for the current population, that is selection, crossover and mutation are applied. When the termination criterion is met, the GA evolution process is terminated and results to one diagnosis classifier for each different diagnosis category.

The objective function estimates the goodness (fitness) of each individual (binary string) and is presented in Figure 11, where *g* is a two-dimension (*m*x22) array representing the *m* genomes of the current population (with 22 genes each representing 22 parameter values), *d* is also a two-dimension (*n*x22) array representing the *n* examples/patterns of the training medical dataset (with 22 parameter values each), *matches* is a counter that counts how many data patterns a gene of the current genome matches, *fitness* is a variable representing the fitness value of the current genome and *limit* is a constant representing the minimum number of matches that a gene must have with the corresponding genes of the patterns of the training dataset to add '1' to its genome's fitness value.

The output for each diagnosis category is a binary string consisting of 22 substrings, each one of which corresponds to a value of a specific parameter denoted by an integer. For example, '2212221111111111133111' is such output for the 'psychogenic' case and constitutes its classifier. In this classifier, the 17th parameter has value '1' (parameter_17 = 1), which corresponds e.g., to the fact "cholesterol is low" ('1' represents 'low').

The rule extraction process is as follows: After the GA evolution process is completed and the classifier for each different diagnosis category is produced, the system tries to identify, for each different classifier, the most important parameters of each diagnosis category. This is done as follows: For each classifier, it tries to find the parameters for which the specific classifier has different values compared to the other three classifiers. For example, the classifier for the psychogenic case has different values compared to the other four classifiers for the parameters in the places 14 (*non-coital*), 15 (*onset*), 17 (*cholesterol*), 18 (*NPT*) and 21 (*DICC*). These five parameters are used in order to construct the final form of the classifier. So, the rule extraction process is able to extract only the important parameters, which are significant for a specific diagnosis category and omit all the others. After that, the execution of another GA, which is designed in order to evolve logical rules, takes place. This GA evolves the set of logical rules corresponding to different combinations of the significant parameters and finally results in the one that better classifies the cases of the training set.

As stated before, REGA is a GA used to evolve the set of symbolic rules corresponding to different combinations of the significant parameters, which have been extracted based on the differences between the diagnosis classifiers. This GA, which is executed one time for each different category, works as follows: It initially creates a set of random logical rules which are combinations of the significant parameter-value pairs extracted. An example of the form of the genomes comprising the GA's population is:

Paramater_17=3 and Parameter_18=3 or Parameter_21=1

Both parameters' relations and logical operators are stored in one-dimensional array.

After the initial population is created, the GA evolves the population of these logical rules by applying genetic operators (crossover, mutation, and selection) and finally, after five generations at most, results in the most appropriate classifying rule for each different category.

The crossover operator used is the classical one-point crossover for one-dimensional array. As a crossover point, only logical operators are selected. The operation of this crossover operator is presented in Figure 12. In that figure, the first logical operator is selected as a crossover point and the parts after this point of both genomes are swapped.

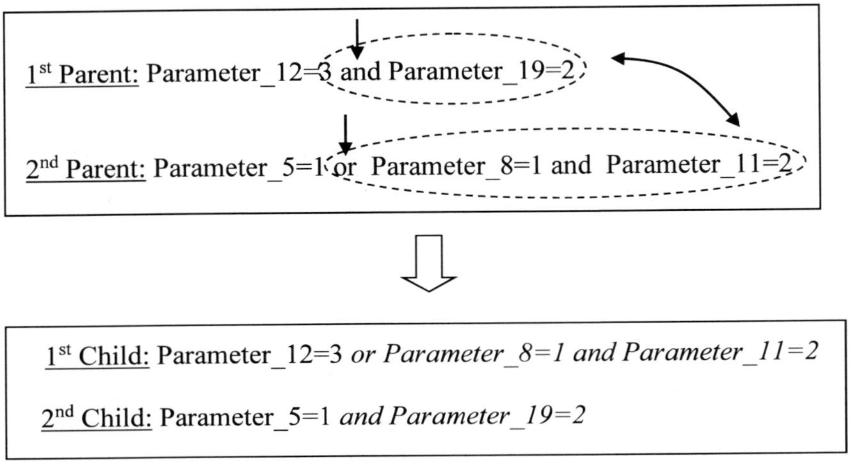

Figure 13. The operation of the crossover operator.

The mutation operator used is the classical swap mutator for one-dimensional array, but it is applied only to logical operators (an 'and' mutates to an 'or' and vice versa). The operation of this mutation operator is presented in Figure 13. In this figure, again the first logical operator is selected for mutation.

The objective function estimates the goodness (fitness) of each individual (logical rule) and is presented in Figure 14, where n is the number of examples/patterns of the training medical dataset and fitness is a variable representing the fitness value of the current genome. We remind that this procedure is executed for each different category.

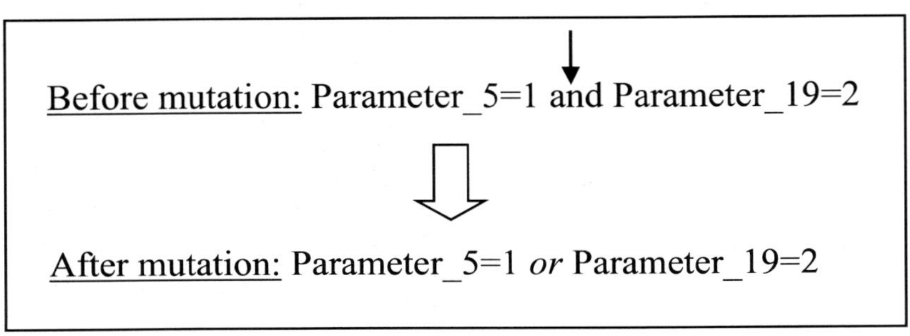

Figure 14. The operation of the mutation operator.

```
fitness = 0;
for i = 1 to n do
    if rule is true
        then fitness =fitness + 1;
    endif
```

Figure 15. Fitness computation.

IMPLEMENTATION DETAILS

The type of the GA used to create diagnosis classifiers is the classic simple GA. The representation used for the genomes of the genetic population is the classic binary string. As far as the reproduction operator is concerned, the classic biased roulette wheel selection is used. The crossover operator used is a uniform crossover (with crossover probability equal to 0.9), while the mutation operator is the flip mutator (with mutation probability equal to 0.001). Except that, the size of the population is set to 50 while the GA uses linear scaling and elitism [27].

The type of the GA used to evolve logical rules is also the classic simple GA. The representation used for the genomes of the genetic population is the one-dimensional array as stated above. As far as the reproduction operator is concerned, the classic biased roulette wheel selection is used. The crossover operator used is the uniform crossover for one-dimensional array (with crossover probability equal to 0.8), while the mutation operator is the swap mutator for one-dimensional array (with mutation probability equal to 0.001 [27]. Except that, the size of the population is set to 10 while the GA uses linear scaling and elitism.

Both GAs was implemented using the C++ Library of Genetic Algorithms GAlib [15]. Especially, the GASimpleGA class was used for the implementation of the GA for creating diagnosis classifiers (non-overlapping populations) and the GABin2DecGenome class for the binary string genomes (an implementation of the traditional method for converting binary strings to decimal values). As far as the GA for evolving logical rules is concerned, the GASimpleGA class was used for its implementation and the GA1DArrayGenome and the GAAlleleSet classes were used for the logical rule's genomes.

The rule-based part of the system has been implemented in CLIPS 6.241 expert system shell.

EXPERIMENTAL RESULTS-PART A

We used for our experiments 700 patient records from the university hospital of Patras. 60% of them (420 cases) were used for training or design purposes. So, we used them for medical knowledge analysis and modeling, for tuning FESMI (e.g specifying membership functions etc) and extracting classifiers and rules in GADIS via the GAs. The rest 40% (280 cases) were used for testing and comparing the two systems.

HISMI: COMBINING FESMI AND GADIS

Each parallel module produced its own diagnosis and an associated reliability value. The latter was a function of the "sensitivity", "specificity" and "accuracy" of the result based on the input-output parameters of a training data set. These typical values were represented by fuzzy sets and the degree to which each patient satisfied the respective diagnosis computed. The overall diagnosis reliability was obtained by considering the conjunction of this constraint satisfaction (i.e., the maximum of the individual reliability values). The final diagnosis value according to the EC rule extraction method took the least time and information but produced the largest error for specific output values. The FESMI approach took the largest time and number of inputs but produced the lowest error, between the two models. However, the fusion of the two models produced the most accurate and reliable results, presented in the next section.

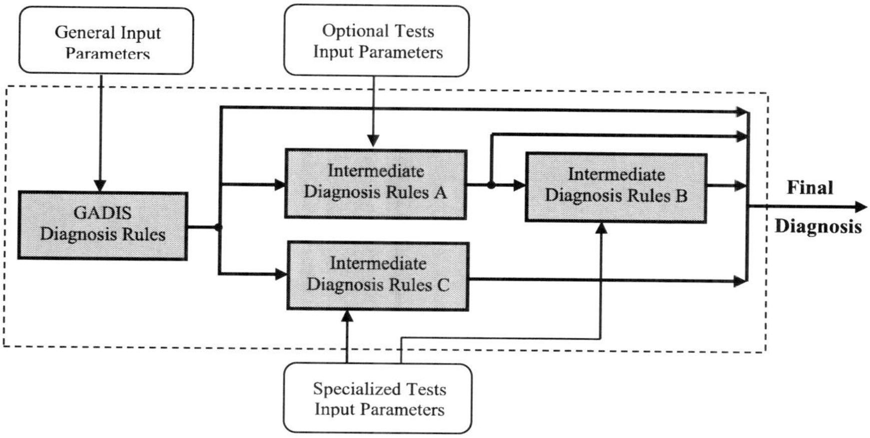

Figure 16. The HISMI final model.

More specifically, the final diagnosis resulted from FESMI and the final diagnosis resulted from the EC module are combined according to their metrics parameters implemented in the formula:

Output = *Final_Diagnosis {max(SensF, SensGA), max(SpesF, SpesGA), max (AccF, AccGA, max (PrecF, PrecGA)}*

where *SensF and SensGA*, are the Sensitivity values from Fuzzy and EC module, *SpesF and SpesGA* are the Specificity values from Fuzzy and EC module, *AccF and AccGA* are the Accuracy values from Fuzzy and EC module and *PrecF and PrecGA* are the Accuracy values from Fuzzy and EC module.

According to this formula and the given data set the system uses FESMI or EC module for different type of final diagnosis to calculate the output value.

EXPERIMENTAL RESULTS

The HDSS under the name HISMI as well as FESMI were run for 350 patient cases, whose records were taken from the hospital database, including 700 records. Their corresponding results were compared both to the results of three urology residents and those of an expert doctor, who is the director of the "Andrology Lab" (Tables 2a, b). As can be easily seen from the tables, the results of FESMI, for each stage of the reasoning process, is quite closer to the expert's than those of the residents (i.e., three different non-expert doctors). For example, FESMI has a 79% success compared to the expert (e.g., see Table 2b, for Psychogenic cases).

We also used the same set to determine the regression coefficients (via SPSS 14.0). Afterward, we applied the remaining patient records, considering them as the test set. We also applied HISMI to the same set of data. In order to evaluate both FESMI and the EC rule generation module and compare their corresponding results, we use three metrics, commonly used for evaluation of predictions: accuracy, sensitivity, specificity and precision (abbreviated as Acc, Sen, Spec, Prec respectively), defined by the following formulas:

$$Acc = (a + d)/(a + b + c + d),$$
$$Sen = a/(a + b),$$
$$Spec = d/(c + d) \text{ and}$$
$$Prec = a/(a+c)$$

Table 2a. Comparison FESMI, GADIS and HISMI (%)

Final Organic Diagnosis	GADIS %	F.E.S.M.I. %	Expert %
Arteriopathy	35	31	30
Venooclusive	15	15	16
Neuropathy	5	5	5
Endocrinopathy	2	2	5

Table 2b. Comparison FESMI, GADIS and HISMI (%)

Possible Diagnosis	GADIS% %	F.E.S.M.I.% %	H.I.S.M.I.% %	Expert %
Psychogenic	49	43	46	47
Organic	51	57	54	53

where *a* is the number of positive (success) cases correctly classified, *b* is the number of positive cases misclassified as negative (fail), *d* is the number of negative cases correctly classified and *c* is the number of negative cases misclassified as positive. Accuracy shows how good the system is in predicting correctly a patient's diagnosis (success or failure). Sensitivity shows how good the system is in predicting success, while specificity shows how good the system is in predicting failure. The evaluation results are presented in Tables 3a, 3b and 3c.

Table 3a. Comparison of FESMI, GADIS and HISMI (accuracy)

POSSIBLE DIAGNOSIS	GADIS	F.E.S.M.I.	H.I.S.M.I.
Psychogenic	0,90	0,84	0,94
Organic	0,83	0,89	0,98
FINAL ORGANIC DIAGNOSIS	**GADIS**	**F.E.S.M.I.**	**H.I.S.M.I.**
Arteriopathy	0,86	0,80	0,86
Venooclusive	0,88	0,88	0,90
Neuropathy	0,94	0,98	1,00
Endocrinopahty	0,98	0,98	1,00

Table 3b. Comparison of FESMI, GADIS and HISMI (sensitivity)

POSSIBLE DIAGNOSIS	GADIS	F.E.S.M.I.	H.I.S.M.I.
Psychogenic	0,88	0,81	0,94
Organic	0,80	0,90	0,98
FINAL DIAGNOSIS	**GADIS**	**F.E.S.M.I.**	**H.I.S.M.I.**
Arteriopathy	0,93	0,90	0,93
Venooclusive	0,80	0,81	0,82
Neuropathy	0,71	1,00	1,00
Endocrinopahty	0,80	0,67	1,00

Table 3c. Comparison of FESMI, GADIS and HISMI (specificity)

POSSIBLE DIAGNOSIS	GADIS	F.E.S.M.I.	H.I.S.M.I.
Psychogenic	0,92	0,86	0,96
Organic	0,87	0,89	0,92
FINAL DIAGNOSIS	**GADIS**	**F.E.S.M.I.**	**H.I.S.M.I.**
Arteriopathy	0,79	0.65	0,79
Venooclusive	0,90	0,91	0,94
Neuropathy	0,98	0,98	1,00
Endocrinopahty	1,00	1,00	1,00

From the results presented in the above tables, someone can come to the conclusion that both HISMI and FESMI achieve about the same accuracy. However, HDSS is more balanced in the Psychogenic final diagnosis as well as in the arteriopathy final diagnosis compared to FESMI, whereas FESMI is more balanced in the venooclusive final diagnosis. This means that it misclassifies more failures than successes, which is not desirable. It is generally preferable to have misclassifications of successes than of failures (it's medically more useful). After the first implementation of the system (Table 2a,b) according to each subsystems' accuracy, real-time diagnosis with new patient data concludes using FESMI Modules' final diagnosis for Organic and EC Modules' final diagnosis for Psychogenic diagnosis. Additionally, after each new diagnosis, the new patient data are added in the systems' database according to the follow up (Figure 14).

Updating the current patient database, the total systems' performance can be altered after the implementation of new tuning procedures, that are programmed to happen after a (total_record_number)*30% new patient entries. Finally, complementary using the two modules of our system in the rest patient records of the hospital database (including 700 records) according to their metrics we have reached a total, mean success of 90% (=mean accuracy) of the expert classification for final diagnosis

CONCLUSION

In this contribution, we presented the design, implementation, and evaluation of HISMI, an intelligent Hybrid medical Decision Support System that deals with the diagnosis of male impotence. The complex systems associated with human activity are often poorly defined. Hybrid computing provides an effective and efficient way to analyze technological processes and human activities. In this work, HDSS is discussed under the aspects of Knowledge Modelling (KM), where the treatment of imprecision is used to explain the reasoning to achieve a conclusion. Fuzzy sets and fuzzy logic can be used to express uncertain information in exact form. The hybridism not only complements the traditional expert systems but also improves the reasoning facilities which is difficult to achieve using a pure EC technique. Using this hybrid system has proved to provide an easier Knowledge Modelling (KM) phase than that expected in KM performed with the use of symbolic techniques alone. Additionally, although the optimization of fuzzy rules in FESMI module achieves an acceptable score, it is necessary to refine them. This refinement is achieved using the EC module. So, the system is capable of translating the encoded knowledge among the various connections between input-output in rules. Besides, all the examples applied in order to test the system's performance demonstrated that the procedure to reduce the number of redundant rules, after the learning and refinement stages of the FESMI, was surprisingly suitable. The domain area applied to validate the HISMI was the classification of impotent males. Experimental results showed that the HISMI performed quite better than a pure fuzzy expert system but worse than the expert. It was also observed that, once again, complex problems as the medical one mentioned in this work are satisfactorily solved by applying hybrid computing.

The future appears to hold a lot of promise for the novel use and combinations of SC applications. The circle of SC's related technologies will probably widen beyond its current constituents. The push for low-cost solutions combined with the need for intelligent tools will result in the deployment of hybrid systems that efficiently more tightly integrate reasoning and search techniques in a single computational unit. Finally, this application will be easily transferred in a mobile system for fast use of residents or even experts that are working in the specific medical field [45].

REFERENCES

[1] Abbod, MF; von Keyserlingk, DG; Linkens, DA; Mahfouf, M. Survey of Utilization of Fuzzy Technology in Medicine and Healthcare, *Fuzzy Sets and Systems*, 120, pp. 331–349, 2001.

[2] Annunziato, M; Lucchetti, M; Pizzuti, S. Adaptive Systems and Evolutionary Neural Networks: a Survey, EUNITE2002, Albufeira, Portugal, Sept. 2002.

[3] Back, T; Fogel, DB; Michalewicz, Z. Handbook of Evolutionary Computation, Bristol, UK: Institute of Physics, and New York, NY: Oxford University Press., (1997).

[4] Bagli, DJ; Agarwal, SK; Venkateswaran, S; Shuckett, B; Khoury, AE; Merguerian, PA; McLorie, GA; Liu, K; Niederberger, CS. Artificial neural networks in pediatric urology: prediction of sonographic outcome following pyeloplasty. *J Urol.*, 1998 Sep, 160(3 Pt 2), 980-3, discussion 994.

[5] Bezdek, J; Dubois, D; Prade, H. (Eds) Fuzzy Sets in Approximate Reasoning and Information Systems (The Handbooks of Fuzzy Sets Series, Fshs 5), Kluwer Academic Publishers., (1999).

[6] Bonissone, PP; Cheetham, W; Golibersuch, D; Khedkar, PS. 'Automated Residential Property Valuation: An Accurate and Reliable Based on Soft Computing', in Soft Computing in Financial Engineering, R. Ribeiro, H. Zimmermann, R. R. Yager, and J. Kacprzyk, Eds., Heidelberg, Germany: Physica-Verlag (Springer-Verlag), 1998.

[7] Bonissone, PP. 'Soft Computing: the Convergence of Emerging Reasoning Technologies', Soft Computing A Fusion of Foundations, *Methodologies and Applications*, 1(1), 6-18, (1997).

[8] Brasil, LM; Azevedo, FM; Barreto, JM. A hybrid expert system for the diagnosis of epileptic crisis, *Artificial Intelligence in Medicine*, No. 585, p. 1-7, (2000).

[9] Chang, PL; Li, YC; Wang, TM; Huang, ST; Hsieh, ML; Tsui, KH. Evaluation of a decision-support system for preoperative staging of prostate cancer. *Med Decis Making*., 1999, Oct-Dec, 19(4), 419-27.

[10] Cordon, O; Herrera, H; Lozano, M. 'A classified review on the combination fuzzy logic-genetic algorithms bibliography', Tech. Report 95129, URL:http://decsai.ugr.s/herrera/flga.html, Department of Computer Science and AI, Universidad de Granada, Granada, Spain, 1995.

[11] Dounias, G. Hybrid Computational Intelligence in Medicine, Workshop in Intelligent and Adaptive Systems in Medicine Prague, March 31 - April 1, (2003).

[12] Dounias, GD; Linkens, DA. (Eds.), Adaptive Systems and Hybrid Computational Intelligence in Medicine, Special Session Proceedings of the EUNITE 2001 Symposium, Tenerife, Spain, December 13-14, 2001, A Publication of the University of the Aegean, ISBN 960-7475-19-4.

[13] Dubois, D; Prade, H. 'Soft computing, fuzzy logic, and Artificial Intelligence', Soft Computing: A Fusion of Foundations, *Methodologies and Applications*, 2(1), 7-11, (1998).

[14] Fogel, DB. Evolutionary Computation: Toward a New Philosophy of Machine Learning, IEEE Press., (1995).

[15] GAlib - A C++ Library of Genetic Algorithm Components, Matthew Wall, Massachusetts Institute of Technology (MIT). Available: http://lancet.mit.edu/ga/.

[16] Gen, M; Cheng, R. Genetic Algorithms and Engineering Design, John Wiley & Sons, Ltd., (1997).

[17] Georgopoulos, E; Likothanassis, S; Adamopoulos, A. 'Evolving Artificial Neural Networks using Genetic Algorithms', International Conference on Artificial Neural Networks and Intelligent Systems (NNW 2000), Prague, Chez Republic, July 9-12, 2000.

[18] Goldberg, DE. Genetic Algorithms in Search, Optimization and Machine Learning, Addison-Wesley, Reading, Mass., (1989).

[19] Hatzilygeroudis, I; Prentzas, J. Knowledge Representation Requirements for Intelligent Tutoring Systems, *Intelligent Tutoring Systems*, pp. 87-97, (2004).

[20] Holland, JH. Adaptation in Natural and Artificial Systems: An Introductory Analysis with Applications to Biology, Control, and Artificial Intelligence, University of Michigan Press (second edition: MIT Press, 1992), (1975).

[21] http://www.ghg.net/clips/CLIPS.html.

[22] http://www.soft-computing.de.

[23] Jardin, A; Wagner, G; Khoury, S; Giuliano, F; Padman Nathan, H. and Rosen R., Erectile Dysfunction, ISSIR, Pr S. Khoury, (Eds) (1999), pp. 115-138.

[24] Fouad R. Kandeel, Vivien K. T. Koussa, Ronald S. *Swerdloff Male Sexual Function and Its Disorders: Physiology, Pathophysiology, Clinical Investigation, and Treatment Endocrine Reviews*, 22 (3), 342-388.

[25] Koutsojannis, C; Hatzilygeroudis, I. *FESMI: A fuzzy expert system for diagnosis and treatment of male impotence Lect Notes Comput Sc*, (2004), 3214, 1106-1113.

[26] Medsker, LR. Hybrid Intelligent Systems, Kluwer Academic Publishers, Boston, 1995.

[27] Michalewicz, Z; Fogel, DB. How to Solve It: Modern Heuristics, Springer-Verlag, Berlin, Heidelberg. (2000).

[28] Michalewicz, Z. Genetic Algorithms + Data Structures = Evolution Programs, Springer-Verlag, Berlin, (1999).

[29] Mitchell, M. An Introduction to Genetic Algorithms, The MIT Press, Cambridge, Massachusetts, London, England., (1996).

[30] Negnevitsky, M. Artificial Intelligence. A guide to Intelligent Systems, 2002, Addison Wesley, ISBN. 0-201-71159-1.

[31] Nguyen, HP; Kreinovich, V. "Fuzzy Logic and Its Applications in Medicine", *International Journal of Medical Informatics*, *62*, pp. 165–173, 2001.

[32] Perimenis, P; Gyftopoulos, K; Giannitsas, K; Markou, SA; Tsota, I; Chrysanthopoulou, A; Athanasopoulos, A; Barbalias, G. A comparative, crossover study of the efficacy and safety of sildenafil and apomorphine in men with evidence of arteriogenic erectile dysfunction. *Int J Impot Res.*, 2004 Jan, 16(1), 2-7.

[33] Perimenis, P; Markou, S; Gyftopoulos, K; Athanasopoulos, A; Giannitsas, K; Barbalias, G. Switching from long-term treatment with self-injections to oral sildenafil in diabetic patients with severe erectile dysfunction. *Eur Urol.*, 2002 Apr, 41(4), 387-91.

[34] Rotshtein, A; Rakytyanska, H. Genetic Algorithm for Fuzzy Logical Equations Solving in Diagnostic Expert Systems, *Lecture Notes in Computer Science*, (2000), Vol. 2070, pp. 349

[35] Schaffer, JD; Whitley, D; Eshelman, LJ. 'Combinations of Genetic Algorithms and Neural Networks: A Survey of the State of the Art', International Workshop on Combinations of Genetic Algorithms and Neural Networks, Baltimore, Maryland, June 6, 1992, pp. 1-37.

[36] Tsakonas, A; Dounias, G. Intelligent Applications - Hybrid Computational Intelligence Schemes in Complex Domains: An Extended Review, in Lecture Notes in Computer Science 2002, Springer Publications, (2002), Vol. 2308, pp. 494 - 512.

[37] Tsakonas, A; Dounias, G; Jantzen, J; Axer, H; Bjerregaard, B; Graf von Keyserlingk, D. Evolving rule-based systems in two medical domains using genetic programming, *Artificial Intelligence in Medicine*, (2004), Vol. 32, Issue 3, pp. 195-216.

[38] Vose, MD. The Simple Genetic Algorithm: Foundations and Theory, MIT Press, (1998).

[39] Wang, ZS; Chen, JDZ. Robust ECG R-R wave peak detection using Evolutionary-Programming-based Fuzzy Inference System (EPFIS) and its application to assessing brain-gut interaction, 1st Int. Conf. on Adv. In *Medical Signal and Inf. Processing*, (IEE Conf. Publ. No. 476), pp. 265-274, (2000).

[40] Whitley, LD. *Foundations of Genetic Algorithms*, 2, Morgan Kaufmann, (1993).

[41] Whitley, LD; Vose, MD. *Foundations of Genetic Algorithms*, 3, Morgan Kaufmann., (1995).

[42] Wu, X; Sharif, BS; Hinton, OR. 'An Improved Resource Allocation Scheme for Plane Cover Multiple Access Using Genetic Algorithm', *IEEE Transactions on Evolutionary Computation*, Vol. 9, No. 1, February 2005.

[43] Zadeh, LA. 'Fuzzy Logic and Soft Computing: Issues, Contentions and Perspectives', in Proc. of IIZUKA'94: Third Int. Conf. on Fuzzy Logic, *Neural Nets and Soft Computing*, 1-2, Iizuka, Japan, 1994.

[44] Zadeh, LA. 'Some reflection on soft computing, granular computing and their roles in the conception, design and utilization of information/intelligent systems', Soft Computing A Fusion of Foundations, *Methodologies and Applications*, 2(1), 23-25, (1998).

[45] Koutsojannis, C; Lithari, C; Hatzilygeroudis, I. Managing urinary incontinence through hand-held real-time decision support aid. *Computer methods and programs in biomedicine*, 03/2012, 107(1), 84-9.

BIOGRAPHICAL SKETCH

Constantinos Koutsojannis

Assoc. Prof. Constantinos Koutsojannis is currently Director of Laboratory of Health Physics & Computational Intelligence, in University of Patras. He is Medical Physicist and expert in Medical Informatics. He is teaching Biophysics, Biostatistics, Research Methodology, Computational Intelligence, Artificial Intelligence and Medical Informatics in several undergraduate and master programs of University of Patras, University of Ioannina and University of Athens. He is involved in a number of Research and Development National and European Projects concerning Artificial Intelligence and serves as a consultant in Artificial Intelligence Working Group as well as full member of Project Committee of European Federation of Medical Physics. His research deals with Biophysics and Medical Applications with Artificial Intelligence on diagnosis, treatment and training using methods of Medical Knowledge representation and extraction from patient data record, medical textbooks and field experts. He has published in a number international journals, conferences and books on the fields of his interest.

Grigorios Beligiannis

Assoc. Prof. Grigorios Beligiannis graduated from the Department of Computer Engineering & Informatics of the University of Patras in 1997. He finished his postgraduate studies in "Computer & Information Technology" in 2000 and his doctoral dissertation in 2002 at the same time Department. In 2007 he was elected to the lecturer's degree with knowledge area "Management Information Systems". In 2011 he has evolved at the rank of Assistant Professor and in 2016 at Associate Professor with subject "Intelligent Information Systems". He has 36 published research papers in international scientific journals and more than 42 published papers in scientific conferences. He is Associate Editor of International Journal of Artificial Intelligence and Member of the Editorial Board of Applied Soft Computing, Helyion, International Journal of Intelligent Information Systems and Artificial Intelligence Research. He has been a member of the Organizing Committee at more than 60 international scientific conferences. His research interests focus on Algorithms of Decision Theory, on Intelligent Algorithm Applications to Operations Research problems and on Business Intelligence Systems.

Ioannis Hatzilygeroudis

Prof. Ioannis Hatzilygeroudis is Professor in the Department of Computer Engineering & Informatics of the University of Patras. He is Associate Editor-in-Chief of the International Journal of Artificial Intelligence Tools (IJAIT). He has also been a member of Program Committees in over 70 international conferences and has organized several invited / special sessions in international conferences. He has published more than 100 scientific papers in international journals, volumes and conference proceedings. He has also participated in a number of National and European projects both as a partner and as a coordinator. She has been teaching programming for over 15 years. His main research interests are: Artificial Intelligence, Knowledge Representation, Knowledge Based /

Experienced Systems, Intelligent Educational Systems and Intelligent E-Learning.

In: Medical Knowledge Extraction … ISBN: 978-1-53617-925-5
Editor: C. M. Koutsojannis

Chapter 9

BIG DATA MINING FOR ANALYSING AND PROCESSING BRAIN SIGNALS HARVESTED WITH SQUID BASED MEG

***Adamantios-Ioannis Statyris[1,*]*,**
Constantinos Koutsojannis[1], PhD
and Ioannis Hatzilygeroudis[2], PhD
[1]Laboratory of Health Physics and Computational Intelligence,
University of Patras, Patras, Greece
[2]Computer Engineering and Informatics Department,
University of Patras, Patras, Greece

ABSTRACT

Studying the human brain has proven to be a difficult task, due to many aspects related to its nature. Its importance as an organ, its complexity in both anatomical and neurophysiological levels, as well as the difficulty presenting due to it being encased in an osseous cavity and of course ethical issues, are some of the most common and important

* Corresponding Author's Email: dr.statiris@gmail.com.

ones. In addition to the aforementioned, brain is a unique organ that encloses a higher level of complexity compared to other organs as its current known primary purpose is to create the perception of life for any individual as a summary of different components deriving from processing all the information that is presented to it by its peripheral sensors and to give them some control to interact with what they eventually perceive as life. In the past, there have been efforts to approach the brain as an object with electrical activity and draw conclusions about its functionality by analysing EEGs. What has been scarcely explored is data from MEGs. SQUID (superconducting quantum interference device) is one of the few magnetometers in the world of exceptionally high capacity to sense minimal Magnetic fields of even the magnitude of 1 fT (10-15 Tesla), electrical currents of 10-18 Amp and voltage of 10-18 Volt, thus we have chosen to analyse data harvested by this device due to its high level of accuracy. The purpose of this work was to exploit two different tools of the field of Artificial Intelligence for knowledge extraction from Big Data, such as classification algorithms, as well as neural networks approach, in order to analyse knowledge related to taste obtained by the 122 lead Magnetometer, SQUID, in order to create an optimal smart system that can predict the taste a subject experiences by analysing the changes in their brain's magnetic signals magnitude and sign.

Keywords: WEKA, neural networks, CLIPS, taste perception, SQUID, magnetometers, taste prediction

INTRODUCTION

Brain Anatomy

In this section we are going to explore the salient anatomical features of the human brain, so as to facilitate the understanding of references to a subgroup of them in the following sections. The brain is an organ encased in the skull, a cavernous bony structure, within which it remains protected, a necessity due to its fragile nature. With the spinal cord traversing all cervical, thoracic and lumbar vertebrae, which constitute the spinal canal, they form the central nervous system (CNS). The bulk of the tissue is made of *grey matter* situated at the *cortex* (outer layer of the brain parenchyma) and of *white* matter forming the inner parts of the brain. These two structures are inverted in the spinal cord levels [1].

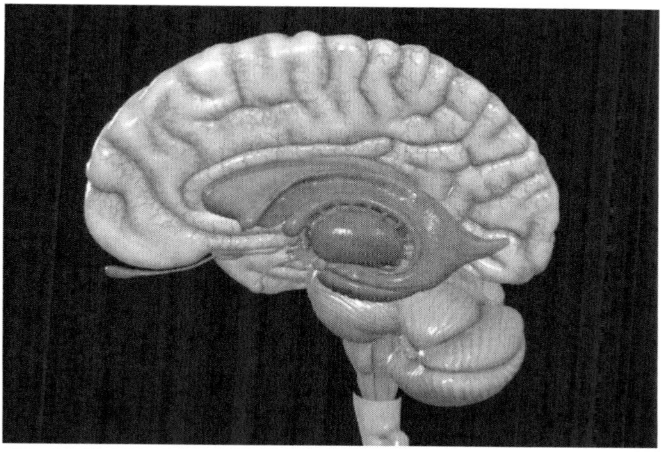

Figure 1. Lateral aspect of the left lateral ventricle: surrounded by the ventricle lies the caudate nucleus (brown) subsequently surrounding the putamen (purple). Covered by the putamen lies first the lateral segment of globus pallidum and closer to the midline, the medial segment. Putamen and the globus pallidum segments form the lentiform nucleus.

Macroscopically the brain consists of 3 elements:

1) The Cerebrum (aka forebrain)
   The cerebrum is the largest part of the brain, and it mainly consists of white and grey matter. Its outer surface is formed by gyri (singular: gyrus), folds of the brain tissue which create indentations of the brain inwards, thus increasing the processing unit of the brain, aka the *Cortex*. The cerebrum consists of two roughly symmetrical hemispheres. In the centre of the two hemispheres, there are two symmetrical cavities, called the lateral ventricles, filled with CSF (cerebro-spinal fluid). Within each of these two ventricles a "choroid plexus" is responsible for all production of this fluid [1]. Following a caudal (downward) direction, the CSF flows through the foramen (hole) of *Monro* to the 3rd ventricle, which rests behind the brain stem and anteriorly to the cerebellum (Figure 7).

2) The cerebellum
   It involves in motor movement, learning repetitive complex movements (i.e.: walking) and is responsible for coordination of fine movements.

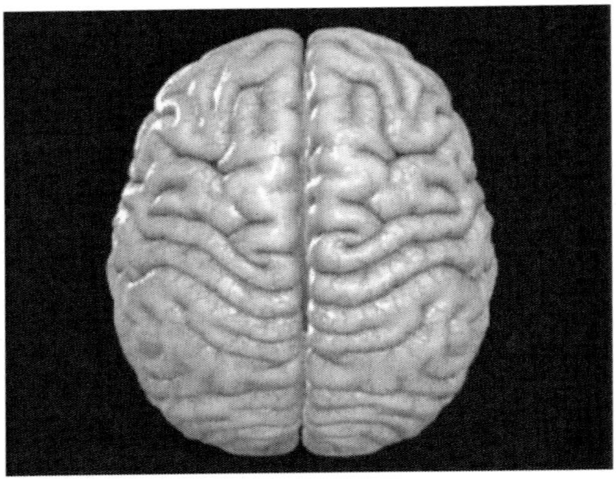

Figure 2. Walnut shaped hemispheres of the brain. R hemisphere on the right side of the image.

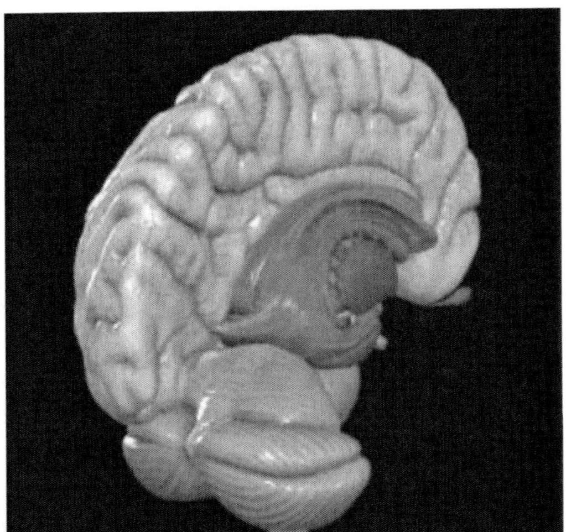

Figure 3. Latero posterior view of the brain missing the R hemisphere. The right-sided lateral ventricle (blue colored) lies in the center of the brain. The cerebellum rests posteriorly under the occipital pole.

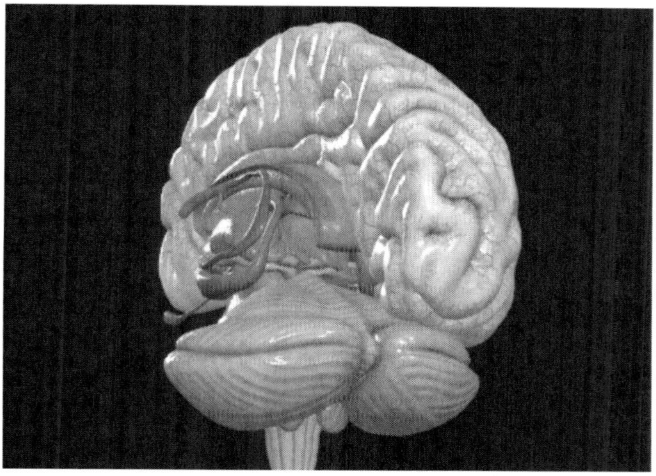

Figure 4. Posterior aspect of the brain (left hemisphere missing), showing the occipital lobe of the brain and the cerebellum (in brown colour) in the lower part of the image.

3) The brainstem (midbrain and hindbrain)

   In the brainstem lie most of the cranial nerves that are involved in functions related to sustaining life, thus their function is tested in brain stem death testing, to declare a patient brain dead [1].

   a) Midbrain:

      Connects the forebrain to the hindbrain. Eye and eyelid movements are controlled by this area of the brain. The midbrain is traversed by the Aqueduct of Sylvius draining the 3rd into the 4th ventricle.

      Cranial Nerves: II, III [1]

   b) Hindbrain:

      I. **Medulla oblongata**: regulates vital involuntary body functions

      II. **Pons**: responsible for sensory analysis, motor control. Involves in sleep and consciousness functions

Cranial nerves: IV, V, VI, VII, VIII, IX, X [1]

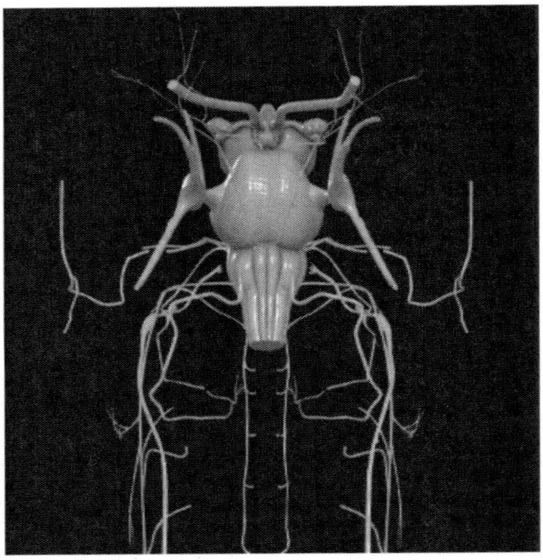

Figure 5. Anterior view of the brain stem and the cranial nerves from underneath. From top to bottom, optic nerves (yellow), amygdales (brown), hypothalamus (light brown), V c. nerve (aka Trigeminal) and its ganglion, stemming out from the pons (light brown bulge). At the lower side of the illustration lies medulla oblongata and the rest of the cranial nerves.

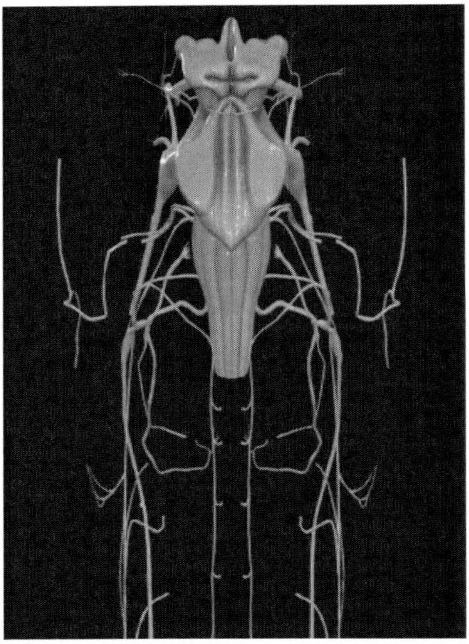

Figure 6. Posterior view of the brain stem and cranial nerves, cerebellum missing.

The CSF Circulation

The brain is a walnut-shaped formation floating inside the skull within a liquid called cerebro-spinal fluid (CSF) and enveloped by three laminae (membranes).

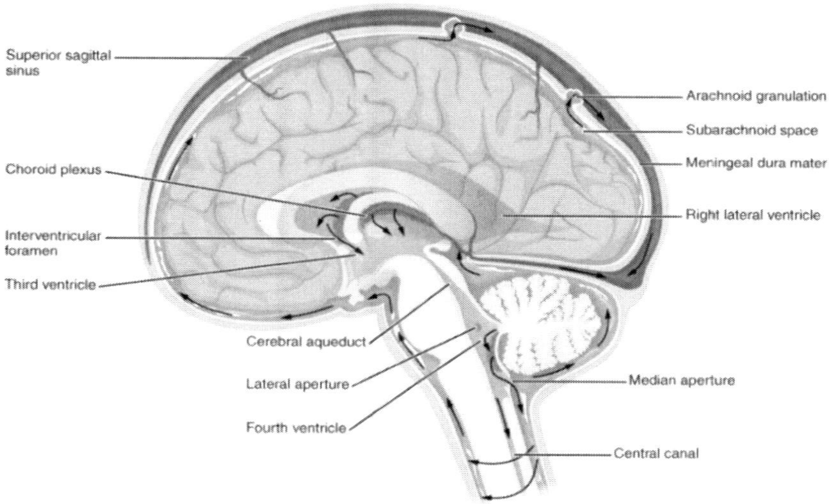

Figure 7. In this illustration, we can easily understand the CSF circulation routes. CSF is produced in the choroid plexuses of the lateral ventricles, flowing to the 3rd ventricle and through the Cerebral aqueduct (aka Aqueduct of Silvius) to the 4th ventricle, immediately anteriorly to the cerebellum. The flow continues divided into two major pathways. One is flowing through the spinal central canal all the way to the caudal part of the spinal cord. In the second pathway, the CSF flows from the 4th ventricle to the cisterns around the brain through the lateral and median apertures, which lay within the 4th ventricle. Subsequently, the CSF will flow in all the subarachnoid spaces, in-between the laminae, reaching the arachnoid granulations in the superior sagittal sinus (one of the largest veins of the brain, resting between the two brain hemispheres), through which it is absorbed in the blood circulation, only to be reproduced later in the choroid plexuses.

Basal Ganglia

The basal ganglia are large stations responsible for regulating all types of gross movements, such as limb movements, facial expressions, and formation of speech. The main groups are, the striatum (part of the forebrain), which consists of the caudate nucleus and the putamen, which accompanied by the globus pallidus' lateral and medial segments all compose the basal ganglia. Furthermore, moving caudally, they interconnect with the thalamic system (part of the forebrain), the subthalamic nucleus and the substantia nigra of the midbrain. In addition, they are in connection with the brainstem in the medulla oblongata, the pons (aka bridge) and the deep cerebellar nuclei [1].

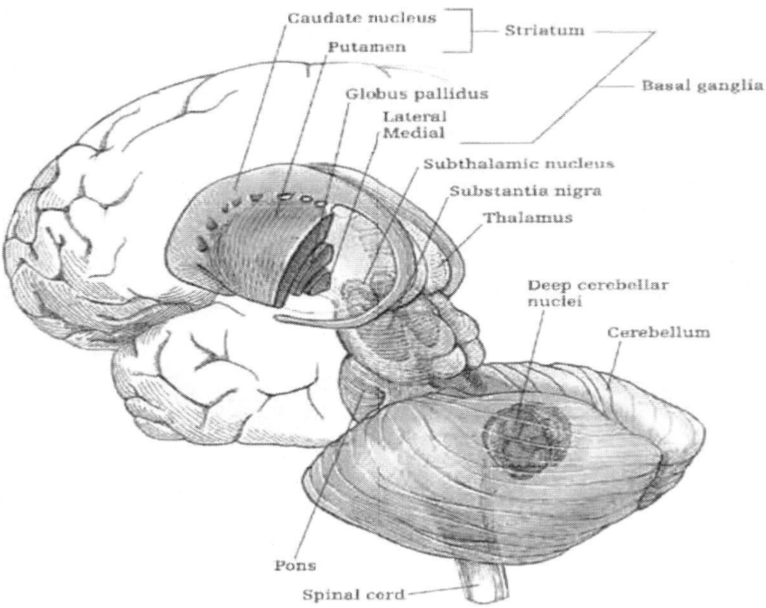

Figure 8. Basal Ganglia, Striatum, Thalamus, Caudate, Putamen, Globus Pallidus, Limbic Striatum, Parkinson's Disease, Alzheimer's Psychosis, Catatonia, Obsessive-Compulsions & Disorders of Movement; Rhawn Gabriel Joseph, Ph.D.; Brain Research Laboratory.

The Cortex

From simple math tasks and color recognition to speech production, recognition, behavioral patterns, music understanding, and poetry, the cortex plays a pivotal role in making what we call subjective reality. The cortex is a vast processing unit of a huge amount of information relayed by the rest of the nervous system, mainly the basal ganglia and some of the brain stem nuclei, and then fed back to them after processing. The neural tissue of the cortex is composed of six layers of primarily neuron cell bodies, unmyelinated axons, dendrites, and synapses, in comparison to white matter which mostly consists of, myelinated long axons. Consensus states that there are roughly about 100 billion neurons in the human brain and each one of them may form up to 15,000 synapses most of which are in the cortex [1].

The subdivides in the frontal, parietal, temporal and occipital lobe. The frontal lobe's margin to the parietal lobe posteriorly is the central sulcus and to the temporal lobe caudally is the *Sylvian* or *lateral sulcus*. Behind the parietal lobe lies the occipital lobe. The *frontal lobe* is largely connected to action; decision making, emotional expression, movement (ocular and skeletal), control of speech and reasoning. A *somatosensory* input is processed in the *parietal lobe*, thus we are able to discriminate two very close separate points on the skin with touch alone. Graphesthesia, and touch localization are other parietal cortical functions. The *temporal lobe* is involved in auditory stimuli relayed directly from the ears and is responsible to translate this information to comprehensible sounds, words, sentences (primary auditory cortex) (left-sided temporal lobe). On the right-sided temporal lobe lies the ability of music comprehension (secondary auditory cortex). It also holds a part in long term *memory* establishment in the hippocampus through amygdala regulation. Other functions of this lobe are naming, verbal memory, object perception and recognition.

Finally, the functions *occipital lobe* serves are related to visual perception in regards to the shape, color, position of an object in space and in time as well. According to A. Faurion et al. fMRI studies have shown that taste signals originating from the gustatory sensors of the tongue predominantly activate the insula of the cortex, an area that is hidden within the Sylvian fissure. This finding is in keeping with the electrophysiological recordings that have been conducted in monkeys, implying gustatory signals are processed in the same cortical area [2]. In addition, a unilateral projection of the inferior part of the dominant hemisphere was noted.

Principles of EEG and MEG

We could describe the brain easily in either anatomical partitions, or less easily in functional areas, yet the most used way of describing the where on the brain with some relative accuracy has been by dividing it based on cytological differences and similarities. In 1909, Brodmann described the cortex of the brain by classifying its areas on cytological criteria. Even though it is not optimal for either research or surgical applications, it has helped us understand the interconnection of different areas of the processing layer of the brain (cortex). This classification has so far been the most widely known, mainly as a useful positioning reference tool. Its major downside, though, is that we can only approximate these areas in live subjects since the area determination process follows histopathologic analysis, thus resection of the brain is necessary. In addition to this, it helps scientists agree with what brain area they are discussing, but only with regards to the cortex, and not in a functional manner. As a result, for the neuroscience to progress into a deep and comprehensive understanding of all the functional, or not, areas of the brain, without being restrained to the surface of it, a new way of studying the brain is needed. Neurosurgery is one of the fields that would benefit greatly from such a breakthrough, since it is of the utmost importance for the surgeon to know exactly what areas are affected and how to approach and resect them in a manner least harmful for other eloquent brain regions. Current practice is far from such a tool, though. Alternatively, so far other approaches have been attempted. The most widely used, even in the daily clinical practice, is the EEG, which can provide information about the electrical activity of the cortex. Another approach has been fMRI, which is invasive and difficult to set up in daily practice, as it involves intravenous contrast and prolonged stillness in an MRI scanner. The contrast might cause an allergy to some subjects, or renal impairment. On top, of these, fMRI provides only crude information, by describing higher blood flows in areas of the brain that are supposedly more active at the time the contrast is injected in the subject. But before we talk about the EEG, we need to talk about the neuron's anatomy, specifically about the neurons of the cortex. They are what we call the *pyramidal neuron*. Pyramidal neurons are neurons with *myelinated* axons. The larger portion of the cell is a triangular like cell body, called *soma* which contains all the basic cell organelles like most other cell types. One side of the body of the cell receives input from small end nerve hair-like terminations, called *(basal) dendrites*. Post-synaptic excitatory and inhibitory potentials meet at the beginning of the thin, long part of the nerve cell called *axon,* and at that area, which is called *hillock*, their nerve cell "decides" whether the summation of the incoming signals will be transferred through the axon to the ending of the nerve terminal *(apical dendrites)* so that it will be transmitted to the next nerve cell. When this happens the membrane of the nerve cell depolarises locally starting from the hillock, which normally rests around roughly -70mV, by opening voltage-gated Na+ ion channels, rushing into the axon, through Na+ ion pumps. The axon is wrapped by myelin layers, which are rich in fatty molecules and electrically isolate the interior of the axon in a way that the ions can only traverse the cell membrane in a few selected regions in between adjacent myelin cells, called Ranvier nodes, which are rich in Na+ ion channels. In this manner when the intracellular environment becomes more positive relatively to the hillock's threshold, it depolarises the membrane locally by opening Na+ ion channels, resulting to bringing more Na+ ions into the cell, as the exterior of the cell is richer in Na+ ions than the interior. The consequent Na+ "excess" triggers the Na+ ion channels in the first Ranvier node, building up even higher levels of Na+ ions, and so on and so forth, thus facilitating the signal to quickly travel across the nerve cell to the nerve terminal [3].

This whole process transforms the nerve cell to be an *electric dipole* for a few moments, being more negatively charged on the body side of the cell, compared to the nerve terminal side. Pyramidal neurons are aligned in a perpendicular manner towards the surface of the brain, with the apical side of the neuron closer to the surface. When an area of the cortex is processing information for a certain purpose, many of these neurons become excited and depolarise, in a way that is largely synchronous, creating a regional current traveling towards the surface of the cortex, which is strong enough to be detected by sensors on the surface of the scalp. EEG is utilizing the physiology of neurons and their ability to create currents vertical to the cortex surface, to record this electrical activity through the skull and the scalp, to study the electrical activity of the brain. It does not come without disadvantages. The biggest one is that information is only obtained by groups of neurons and that only those which are perpendicular to the skull surface. Furthermore, these neurons must be relatively close to the surface, so deep brain area activity cannot be measured, and even for cortex neuron activity, the signals are strong enough to be detected only when thousands of neurons work in synchronicity and adequately close to each other. It is easy for someone to surmise that despite EEG can provide much information about the cortical activity (only), it is still far from accurate spatially. EEG accuracy can be increased if the recording leads are placed directly into the brain's parenchyma, which is an invasive technique, thus involving many risks for unwanted complications [3].

All the neurons in the brain either create, contribute to or relay a signal with or without processing it in the meantime. As it is known from physics every charge movement creates a magnetic field with the direction indicated by the right-hand rule. Thus, the pyramidal neurons of the cortex produce minuscule magnetic fields when they transmit signals from their somas through the axons to their nerve terminals, of the order of the femto- to pico-Tesla.

MEG is the method with which we can observe brain activity by recording the magnetic fields produced into the neurons (on intracellular level). The skull, CSF and other tissues are not interfering with the magnetic fields' strength, thus the magnetic fields can be recorded by extra cranial sensors, called magnetometers and/or gradiometers. Magnetometers are more suitable for detecting deep brain magnetic fields, due to their higher sensitivity to detect magnetic fields, while gradiometers (planar and axial) are more suitable to provide clearer signals since they can filter out most of the ambient noise originating in the Earth's and surrounding electronic devices magnetic fields.

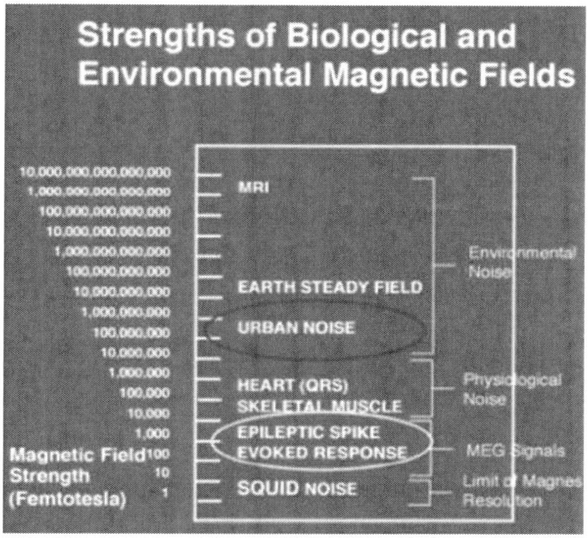

Figure 9. Relative magnetic field magnitudes in femtoTeslas, from SQUID noise to MRI scanner.

MEG is always paired with magnetic resonance imaging (MRI) to compose the Magnetic Source Imaging. MSI can correlate raw MEG recordings to MRI recordings, thus providing high accuracy anatomical positioning, very commonly used in epilepsy surgery or preoperative brain mapping [4].

There are a few differences that bring MEG to an advantageous position compared to EEG regarding their ability for accurate recordings. First and foremost is MEG's ability to detect cortical signals with much higher spatial and temporal accuracy than EEG. Since magnetic fields do not attenuate traversing through human tissue, the recordings coming from areas relatively close to the scalp (neo cortex), are detected with no signal loss, from intracellular currents, whereas the recordings from an EEG come derive from intercellular neuronic activity, after some signal loss occurs due to the human tissue's resistance to current movement.

The second most important difference is that EEGs detect radial currents' activity, in other words, currents with a direction perpendicular to the scalp. MEGs detect tangential signals to the skull surface. This is because according to the right-hand rule, magnetic fields created by radially traveling signals remain inside the skull. Furthermore, MEG needs 3-4 cm^2 of synchronous cortical epileptic activity to be able to detect neural activity. EEG needs 6-20 cm^2. All the above reasons, in parallel to a requirement for high accuracy and detailed source recording, led us to choose MEG over EEG studies for conducting our research on creating a smart system that would mine data good enough for it to be able to pinpoint the salient brain areas that are involved in the taste circuit as we will explore in later sections [4].

SQUID

In essence, Superconducting Quantum Interference Device technology is utilized by magnetoencephalographs (MEGs) employing SQUIDs' high sensitivity to detect very low strength magn etic fields, of the magnitude of 1,000 to 10,000 femtoT. These devices are based on the Josephson Junctions (JJ) which are exploiting the Quantum Tunnelling effect of Cooper electron pairs, which presents on conducting materials that are frozen down to less than a crucial temperature. The Cooper electron pairs start to emerge under that T_c, converting the material into a superconductor. At this state, the material is a perfect diamagnet and there is no electrical resistance at all, enabling current to be created within the material without any voltage requirement. The explanation of these phenomena is related to the *Cooper electron pairs.* A large component of SQUIDs' hypersensitivity to measure subtle magnetic fields is based on the Bardeen, Cooper, Schrieffer theory (BCS). The *BCS theory* states that the electrons involved in converting a conductor to a superconductor are Copper electrons. These are electron pairs that their Fermi level is close enough, such as, in an adequately low temperature ($<T_c$) the kinetic agitation of the subatomic particles is so small that they (the electrons)

develop very weak attraction bonds and they then function as one new active particle with total spin of 0, the *Cooper pair*. At T_c their density is 0, and it increases as the T approaches absolute 0. The second reason for their high sensitivity is the use of 1st and/or 2nd order axial gradiometers in conjunction with planar gradiometers, resulting in filtering out the ambient magnetic noise [5].

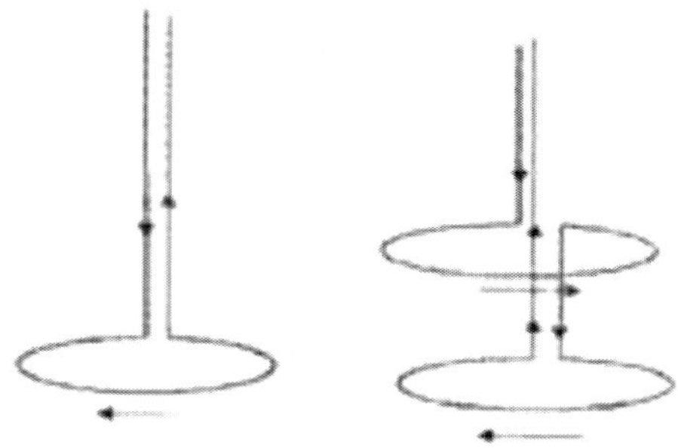

Figure 10. Magnetometer (Left); 1st order axial gradiometer (Right).

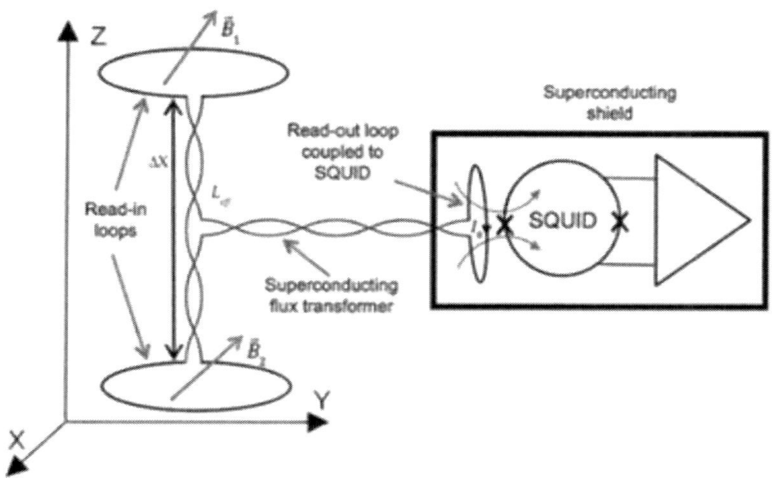

Figure 11. Gravity, Magnetic and Electromagnetic Gradiometry; Strategic technologies in the 21st century; Magnetic gradiometry; Alexey V Veryaskin; Published February 2018 • Copyright © 2018 Morgan & Claypool Publishers; Pages 2-1 to 2-19.

Magnitometers are simple paramagnetic coils that can detect the amplitude of a magnetic field. Their disadvantage is that their disability to distinguish between useful (wanted) input and ambient magnetic noise that derives from the Earth's magnetic field, or electrical or magnetic devices.

Gradiometers, on the other hand, are two (or more) coils in conjunction, in a way that one of them is close to the area of interest and the other one is far away enough so as to function as a point of reference for the ambient magnetic noise in order for it to be canceled out, leaving as net output only the magnitude of the magnetic field that the area of interest is producing [5].

Challenges

Due to the miniscule magnitude of the neurons' magnetic fields, the method of using gradiometers seems inadequate to filter out all the noise. This constitutes one of the greatest engineering problems of a SQUID for brain studies and the solution to it is to encase MEG, SQUIDs, and subject under study into a magnetically shielded room (Faraday Cage).

Furthermore, the technical challenge of the BCS theory to be implemented into SQUIDs is that the whole system needs to be frozen down to a temperature close to 0 °K (absolute zero). This translates into a requirement to construct a thermos for encasing the entire MEG/SQUID system in liquid Helium which is constantly being cooled, otherwise, the phenomenon seizes to exist. Subsequently, one more technical challenge emerges, albeit secondary, that of constructing a thermos in the suitable shape for the type of the area to be studied, as magnetic fields decay quickly with distance, thus the sensors need to be relatively close to the organ under inspection.

Structure

The general structure of a MEG/SQUID system requires a probing end, the SQUIDs, both of which are encased in a thermos, the SQUID electronics and the data acquiring and processing unit.

The probe consists of the sensors which usually are gradiometers that are connected to the SQUID loops via magnetic induction. The superconducting material needs to be sunk into liquid Helium and be frozen down to 0 °K, thus all the aforementioned components of the device are in a thermally insulated thermos.

Then the SQUIDs are connected externally to an information-gathering device such as a computer recording the magnetic activity from the surface of the cerebral cortex for further processing and utilization.

The MEG used in the experiment we are about to explore in the next sections is a 122 channel dcSQUID magnetoencephalography, each channel consisting of a gradiometer and a SQUID device. A dcSQUID converts magnetic flux to a voltage by utilizing a superconducting loop separated by 2 insulators as illustrated in the following picture [6].

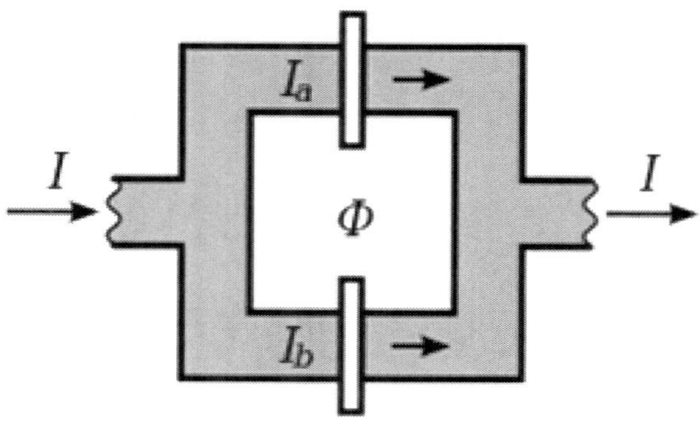

Figure 12. dcSQUID loop illustration;
https://en.wikipedia.org/wiki/SQUID#Cold_dark_matter.

Material and Methods

Taste Dataset from SQUID

SQUIDs initially detect minute magnetic fields produced by pyramidal neurons of the brain. These are detected via the phenomenon of magnetic induction in conjunction with the hypersensitivity provided by the physics of hyperconductivity in low temperatures. Then the magnetic field is converted into electrical current in the coils of the gradiometers/magnetometers, which then is recorded as a temporal array of voltages for each one of the SQUID probes [7, 8, 9, 10]. In this work we have based our study on the data sample collected by Mr Gemousakakis in his work, [6]. For Mr Gemousakakis' PhD, Neuromag-122 was employed to conduct the experiment he had designed. During his study a total of 41 healthy subjects (14 men, 27 women) participated in the experiment, during which they were tested in five different water solutions, of sweet, salty, sour, bitter taste and a control solution which was consisted only of water. They were given a standardised amount of 0.07gr/ml of the gustatory stimulating agent which is considered as an adequate concentration and amount to produce a significant response according to international literature. Thus, 0.07gr/ml sugar and water were given for the sweet taste (SW), 0.07gr/ml of coffee and water for the bitter taste (BT), 0.07gr/ml of lemon juice and water for the Sour Taste (SR) and finally 0.07gr/ml of salt and water for the salty taste (SLT). The first solution given was plain water as a control sample. All the subjects drunk 50ml of each one of these solutions with time intervals of at least 30' in-between the administration. All the MEG recordings would start 2' after the consumption of each of the solutions for every subject.

During our approach to manipulate Gemousakakis' measurements we have chosen to ignore his results so as we would be unbiased by his interpretations. Subsequently, we have only used the recordings made available to us and have created our dataset for pre-processing prior to commencing our study [6].

Our dataset is a derivative stemming from an initial dataset of 41 volunteers, 27 women and 14 men between 9-50 years old. Each individual was defined by 125 attributes (sex, age, taste given, 122 SQUID leads). Because the given tastes were 5 (normal, sweet, salty, sour, bitter), the data set eventually presented with 41 volunteers x5 to end up with a table of 205 entries defined by 125 attributes.

Subsequently, all the subjects of age 18 years or less were removed from the dataset, as Gemousakakis et al. have discovered that there is no significant differentiation in neural response for a taste before the end of adolescence.

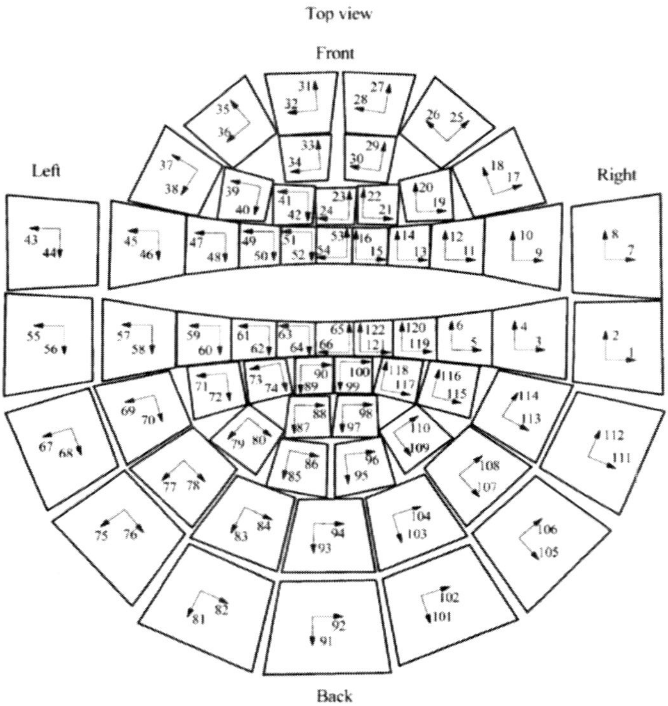

Figure 13. Scan order of the channels; the order into which the channels are read into the memory of the computer. (Neuromag-122 User's Manual: System Hardware).

Furthermore, the sex attribute was removed, since after initial investigation with multiple different tools and sorting algorithms in WEKA (J48 and RandomForest) we could not yield any meaningful results, which was in some significant extent corroborated by Gemousakakis et al. who stated that there are some significant differences in responses in the female subgroup for the tastes of sweet and bitter, but not for the rest [6].

Lastly, Dr Gemousakakis et al. had documented the frequency of 122 different areas of the brain with the aid of SQUID as absolute values. Despite the fact that in their experiment they standardized the procedure of tasting, offering flavours to the volunteers according to a protocol devised (and described earlier), there was no way to have a point of reference between the initial state of mind of the subject during the tasting of the "normal" taste as opposed to the one they had during any other taste they would experience later in the experiment. Thus, in an effort to minimize the "noise" of other cerebral processes (irrelevant to the thoughts of the taste), we subtracted the documented frequencies (2-7Hz) in each end state (sweet, salty, sour, bitter) from the initial state (normal taste) for each individual.

The resulting dataset consisted of 148 entries, each one defined by 123 attributes (122 SQUID leads, taste given), but the SQUID data was the relevant change Hz for each lead, with values of -5, -4, -3, -2, -1, 0, +1, +2, +3, +4, +5, with the sign representing whether the frequency of any given cortical area had increased or decreased due after the taste stimulus was administered.

Data Mining (Decision Trees) Approach

WEKA is a set of tools used for data mining. It contains multiple information extracting algorithms and other tools for the preparation of a data set, classification, clustering, association rules mining and visualizing the mined data [11]. WEKA uses algorithms to pass through data in forms of tables and find associations between the pieces of data to eventually propose a possible sorting of the data, with some similar features, in other words it tries to propose more meaningful ways to view the dataset for the user (Figure 14). The algorithm that we have used in this approach is *J48*. Which is a java implementation of the *C4.5* algorithm, which is used to generate *decision trees*. The reason why we selected this algorithm as most suitable to use in this project is that it has been widely know as a powerful algorithm for creating decision trees, and even stated as the machine learning workhorse most widely used in practice to date in 2011 by the WEKA team. It has also ranked #1 in the survey article *Top 10 Algorithms in data mining in 2007* [12].

J48's most paramount feature is its capability to create a decision tree, which for us would be the backbone of coding our rules in CLIPS, see relevant section. It has been important for our team in this project to try and rely as less as possible on previous anatomical and physiological knowledge about specific areas that might be involved in gustatory perception, for the purpose of revealing AI systems' extent of capability to discover them relying as much as possible on a carefully selected dataset alone (Figure 15).

```
Correctly Classified Instances         122               82.4324 %
Incorrectly Classified Instances        26               17.5676 %
Kappa statistic                          0.7654
Mean absolute error                      0.1068
Root mean squared error                  0.231
Relative absolute error                 28.4752 %
Root relative squared error             53.3631 %
Coverage of cases (0.95 level)         100      %
Mean rel. region size (0.95 level)      35.6955 %
Total Number of Instances              148

=== Detailed Accuracy By Class ===

                 TP Rate  FP Rate  Precision  Recall   F-Measure  MCC      ROC Area  PRC Area  Class
                 0,895    0,091    0,773      0,773    0,773      0,768    0,974     0,907     SW
                 0,868    0,082    0,786      0,786    0,786      0,762    0,971     0,901     SLT
                 0,861    0,045    0,861      0,861    0,861      0,816    0,984     0,945     BT
                 0,663    0,018    0,923      0,923    0,923      0,731    0,969     0,897     SR
Weighted Avg.    0,824    0,060    0,834      0,824    0,823      0,769    0,975     0,912

=== Confusion Matrix ===

  a  b  c  d   <-- classified as
 34  2  1  1 |  a = SW
  2 33  2  1 |  b = SLT
  3  2 21  0 |  c = BT
  5  5  2 34 |  d = SR
```

Figure 14. J48 Algorithm classification results.

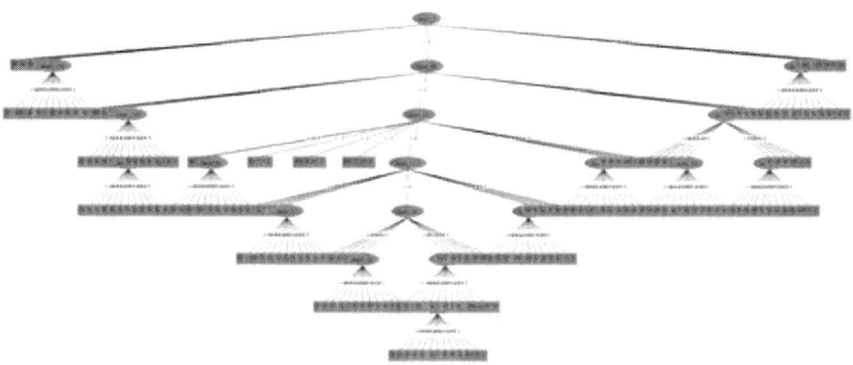

Figure 15. WEKA J48 Decision Tree output.

Machine Learning (Artificial Neural Networks) Approach

Artificial Neural networks are artificially designed computing models created imitating the brain neuronal networks. They can be trained to perform a certain task, recognise patterns in big datasets, classify data and predict future outcomes based on their educated assumptions. They are layered structures of processing, comprising of an input and an output layer and "*hidden*" layers in between them, which can be connected in a linear or non-linear way. Each layer consists of weighted nodes, in which the data is processed in an abstract manner using regression [13]. The network trains itself in a loop, accepting the input in the input layer, processing all the training dataset through the hidden layers and comparing the output to the desired parameters that are defined by the user. The loop repeats, retraining the network, improving each time, aiming to reach a state in which the network can have an acceptable/desired output. Subsequently, this trained Neural Network can be used for predictions regarding the phenomenon studied by the original dataset. Wide used applications of neural networks are applications like facial recognition software, stock market trends, personalised advertising, voice-controlled devices, guidance and navigation etc [14].

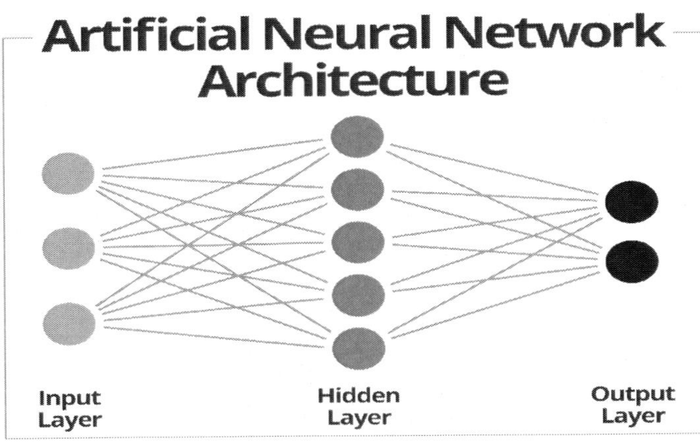

Figure 16. Illustration of a basic Artificial Neural Network (ANN).

Using artificial neural networks we resulted lower level accuracy. After pre-processing and dividing data set to Training, Validation and Test subdatasets [16], the usable dataset became too small for ANNs. The detailed results are presented in Figure 16.

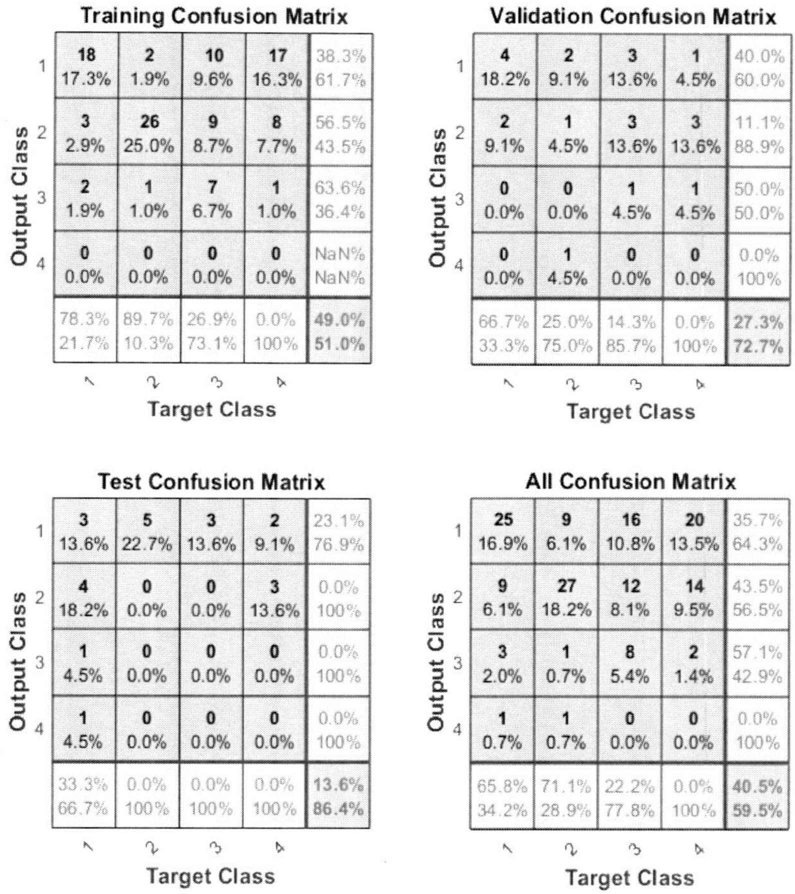

Figure 17. Neural Networks classification results.

DISCUSSION

Even this novel approach in Big Data applications, according to the results there is a need for a repeat with a larger dataset of contributing volunteers of different age sex and race. Moreover, prior to this new endeavour, it is crucial to redesign this the experiment focused on the purpose of this study [17].

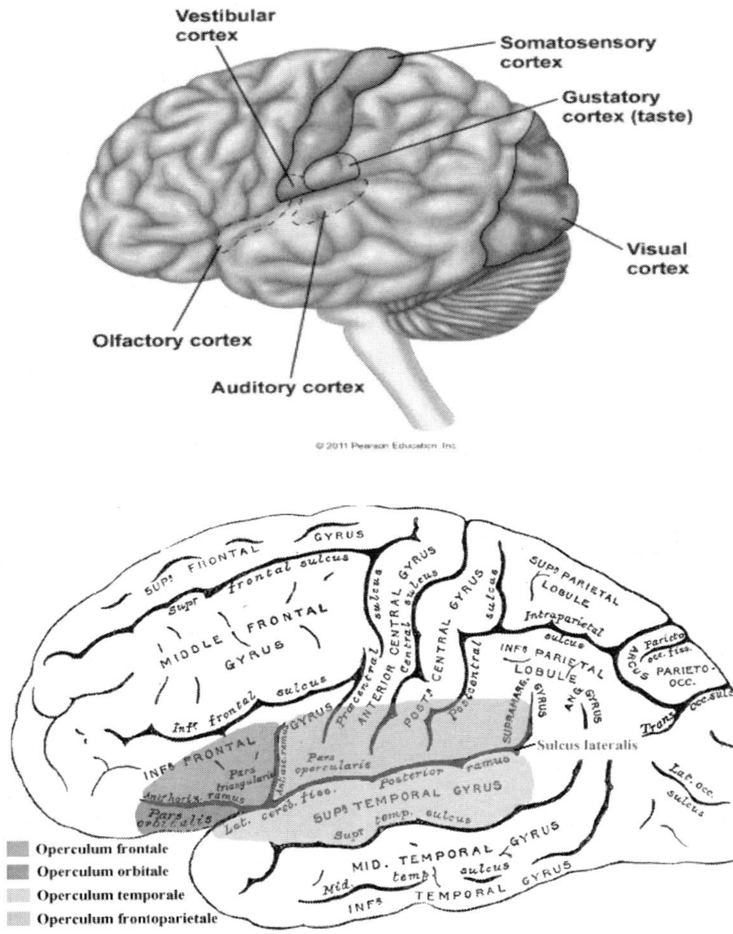

Figure 18. Gustatory cortex (left); Operculum frontale (right). Known areas for gustatory perception so far [1, 6, 17].

According to existing literature, only the anterior insula on the insular lobe and the frontal operculum on the inferior frontal gyrus of the frontal lobe are involved in the perception of taste [1, 6, 17]. Our results derived from J48 in WEKA are indicative of many more areas of the brain to be involved in the process of the gustatory perception, before the brain decides what is the gustatory nature of any given stimulus. One weak point of the study is that the original experiment has no accurate correlation of the MEG leads with specific anatomical structures of the cortex, thus, although we have resulted in suspecting many more cortical areas of the brain, which approximately lie in the areas of the salient nodes of the gustatory network as shown in Figure 19, we have no way of pinpointing them to exact cortical features. For this, redesigning the data collection utilising the application of superimposed fine cut MRI stealth with fiducials prior to entering the tasting phase while subjects are in the SQUID, could dramatically improve the correlation of any results to very specific areas of the cortex.

The following picture illustrates in colour the areas (leads) of the cortex that are possibly involved in the perception of taste. The colours are indicative to what is the majority of the taste perceived (majority defined as half or more of the possible decisions the network made in the last step to decide what was the taste initial stimulus, for every Df [-5,+5]), given the fact that that specific brain area ends up being indeed activated in the taste neural network (Figure 18):

- Predominantly sweet: *red*,
- Predominantly salty: *yellow*,
- Predominantly sour: *lime*,
- Predominantly bitter: *purple* [17].

This is the most important finding of our study, providing new direction to the basic research in the field of neuronal connections and signal sequences in understanding the field of human senses.

The discrepancy between WEKA results with J48 and the ANN approach, is explained due to the fact that as stated earlier, the dataset became eventually small enough to require training and testing on the whole dataset both, which for WEKA and J48 approach would be expected to conclude with good results. Conversely, for the ANN approach, the training, validation and testing subdatasets are mandatorily partitions of the original dataset (which was already shortened in the preprocessing phase), thus resulting to even smaller dataset for the ANN to train upon, which as well was expected to yield low accuracy results. It is well known that the

ANN based systems produce good results when they manage big data. For this reason it is crucial to repeat the experiment with a much larger dataset.

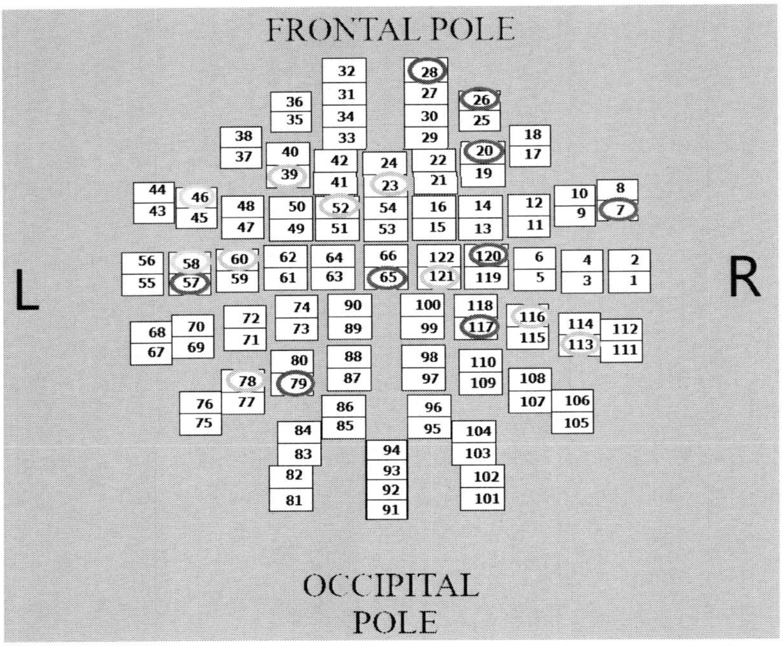

Figure 19. Colour representation of Neural Networks of taste.

CONCLUSION

Using artificial intelligence tools in clinical practice can prove to be beneficial as it could make it easier for health professionals to make useful and informed medical decisions faster and simpler using mobile applications. Understanding the neural network of taste is open and very challenging in the medical and research community. Data mining, and Artificial Intelligence more generally, with the ability to deal with Big Data, is a promising approach [13]. The need for redesigning the experiment in order to verify newly discovered areas as being involved in the gustatory cortical network is the most important related to basic research in this field (Figure 19). Additionally, further implementation of this approach to the other senses, is also desirable, a study that could aspire in revolutionising telecommunications and human-machine interfaces in the medical, industrial fields and everyday life alike. Finally, in the near future and after collecting a richer patient record set the system can update the internal reasoning model, re-calculate its "*new performance and give even more accurate results.*"

REFERENCES

[1] Nguyen, Thai (2010) "Total Number of Synapses in the Adult Human Neocortex," *Undergraduate Journal of Mathematical Modeling: One + Two:* Vol. 3: Iss. 1, Article 14.

[2] Faurion, A, Cerf, B, Van De Moortele, PF, Lobel, E, MacLeod, P, Le Bihan, D; *Neuroscience Letters Volume* 277, Issue 3, 31 December 1999, Pages 189-192.

[3] Britton JW, Frey LC, Hopp JLet al., authors; St. Louis EK, Frey LC, editors. Electroencephalography (EEG): An Introductory Text and Atlas of Normal and Abnormal Findings in Adults, Children, and Infants. Chicago: American Epilepsy Society; 2016.

[4] Singh SP. Magnetoencephalography: Basic principles. *Ann Indian Acad Neurol.* 2014;17(Suppl 1):S107–S112.

[5] Gravity, Magnetic and Electromagnetic Gradiometry; Strategic technologies in the 21st century; Magnetic gradiometry; Alexey V Veryaskin; Published February (2018) Eds, Morgan & Claypool Publishers; Pages 2-1 to 2-19.

[6] Gemousakakis T, Kotini A, Anninos P, Zissimopoulos A, Prassopoulos P. *MEG evaluation of taste by gender difference*. J Integr Neurosci 2011; 10: 537–45.

[7] Anninos PA, Tsagas N, Sandyk R, Derpapas K. *Magnetic stimulation in the treatment of partial seizures. Int J Neurosci.* 1991 Oct;60(3-4):141-7.

[8] Kotini A, Anninos PA, Adamopoulos A, Koutlaki N, Galazios G, Anastasiadis P. Fetal magnetocardiogram recordings and power

spectra analysis in biomagnetic arrhythmic signals. *J Obstet Gynaecol.* 2001 Jul;21(4):368-72.

[9] Kotini A, Anninos P, Adamopoulos A, Prassopoulos P. Low-frequency MEG activity and MRI evaluation in Parkinson's disease, *Brain topography* (2005) 18 (1), 59-63.

[10] Simopoulos C, Anninos P, Polychronidis A, Kotini A, Adamopoulos A. Pre-and postsurgical biomagnetic activity in MALT-type gastric lesions: A case report, *Acta Radiologica* (2003) 44 (2), 154-157.

[11] Hall, Mark, Eibe Frank, Geoffrey Holmes, Bernhard Pfahringer, Peter Reutemann, and Ian H. Witten (2009). The WEKA Data Mining Software: An Update. SIGKDD Explorations, Volume 11, Issue 1.

[12] Xindong Wu, Vipin Kumar, J. Ross Quinlan, Joydeep Ghosh, Qiang Yang, Hiroshi Motoda, Geoffrey J. McLachlan, Angus Ng, Bing Liu, Philip S. Yu, Zhi-Hua Zhou, Michael Steinbach, David J. Hand, Steinberg, Dan, *Top 10 algorithms in data mining*, 2007.

[13] Sarfi, Robert J., A. M. G. Solo, Development of a Hybrid Knowledge-Based System for Multiobjective Optimization of Power Distribution System Operations, 2004, IAAI-05.

[14] Giarratano, Joseph C., Gary D. Riley, Expert Systems: Principles and Programming, 4th Edition, 2004.

[15] MATLAB. https://ch.mathworks.com/discovery/neural-network.html.

[16] Gemousakakis T, Anninos P, Zissimopoulos A. A study on the age dependency of gustatory states: Low-frequency spectral component in the resting-state MEG. *J Integr Neurosci* 2013; 12: 1–13.

BIOGRAPHICAL SKETCHES

Adamantios Ioannis Statyris

Dr Adamantios Ioannis Statyris, currently is training in neurosurgery in King's College Hospital, in London. Initially, he started his surgical career in Patra, Greece. Subsequently he moved to the UK, to continue his training in Neurosurgery. Being a post graduate of the Nursing faculty of the National and Kapodistrian University of Athens, Greece, and while still being an undergrad in Medicine, in the University of Patras, Greece, he undertook a masters in Neuroinformatics. Most points of his thesis are presented in this very chapter. During the last two years, he had been employed by the National Hospital for Neurology and Neurosurgery in the UCLH Trust in London, UK, as a Neurosurgical trainee, both on ward based care and Neurocritical Care alike. During his service in the latter, he has participated in several medical informatics projects for Quality Improvement on behalf of the Neurocritical Care Department (SITU, HDU, MITU, M-HDU). He has always taken a deep interest in the field of Neurosciences and Informatics, and alongside his career in Neurosurgery he aspires to combine all the aforementioned fields to the benefit of patients and everyday technology users alike, utilizing applications in Neuroinformatics to improve healthcare standards and with the view to establish seamless machine-human interface.

Constantinos Koutsojannis

Associate Professor, Constantinos Koutsojannis is currently Director of Laboratory of Health Physics & Computational Intelligence, in University of Patras. He is Medical Physicist and expert in Medical Informatics. He is teaching Biophysics, Biostatistics, Research Methodology, Computational Intelligence, Artificial Intelligence and Medical Informatics in several undergraduate and master programs of University of Patras, University of Ioannina and University of Athens. He is involved in a number of Research and Development National and European Projects concerning Artificial Intelligence and serves as a consultant in Artificial Intelligence Working Group as well as full member of Project Committee of European Federation of Medical Physics. His research deals with Biophysics and Medical Applications with Artificial Intelligence on diagnosis, treatment and training using methods of Medical Knowledge representation and extraction from patient data record, medical textbooks and field experts. He has published in a number international journals, conferences and books on the fields of his interest.

Ioannis Hatzilygeroudis

Dr. Ioannis Hatzilygeroudis is Professor in the Department of Computer Engineering & Informatics of the University of Patras. He is Associate Editor-in-Chief of the International Journal of Artificial Intelligence Tools (IJAIT). He has also been a member of Program Committees in over 70 international conferences and has organized several invited / special sessions in international conferences. He has published more than 100 scientific papers in international journals, volumes and conference proceedings. He has also participated in a number of National and European projects both as a partner and as a coordinator. She has been teaching programming for over 15 years. His main research interests are: Artificial Intelligence, Knowledge Representation, Knowledge Based / Experienced Systems, Intelligent Educational Systems and Intelligent E-Learning.

About the Editor

Constantinos Koutsojannis
Associate Professor
University Of Patras

Associate Professor Constantinos Koutsojannis is currently Director of Laboratory of Health Physics & Computational Intelligence, in University of Patras. He is Medical Physicist and expert in Medical Informatics. He is teaching Biophysics, Biostatistics, Research Methodology, Computational Intelligence, Artificial Intelligence and Medical Informatics in several Undergraduate and Master programs of University of Patras, University of Ioannina and University of Athens. He is involved in a number of Research and Development National and European Projects concerning Artificial Intelligence and serves as a consultant in Artificial Intelligence Working Group as well as full member of Project Committee of European Federation of Medical Physics. His research deals with Biophysics and Medical Applications with Artificial Intelligence on diagnosis, treatment and training using methods of Medical Knowledge representation and extraction from patient data record, medical textbooks and field experts. He has published in a number international journals, conferences and books on the fields of his interest.

INDEX

A

B

C

D

E

F

G

H

I

K

L

M

N

O

P

Q

R

S

T

U

V

W

X

Y